Flanging Techniques in Anterior Segment Surgery

Michael Amon

Editor

Flanging Techniques in Anterior Segment Surgery

Mastering Aphakia, IOL-exchange and IOL-refixation

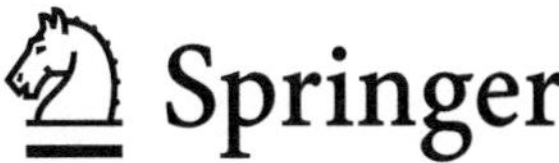 Springer

Editor
Michael Amon
Sigmund Freud University
Vienna, Austria

Department of Ophthalmology
Academic Teaching Hospital of St. John
Vienna, Austria

ISBN 978-3-031-32857-2   ISBN 978-3-031-32855-8   (eBook)
https://doi.org/10.1007/978-3-031-32855-8

This Springer imprint is published by the registered company Springer Nature Switzerland AG
The registered company address is: Gewerbestrasse 11, 6330 Cham, Switzerland

Preface

Progress is not a linear ascending function, but a wave-shaped ascending curve. After times of frustrating work, sudden success makes us jump into the next level of progress. From this level, with hard labor and with a huge time investment, we again will find solutions for further progress, sometimes after a period of detour or even regression Fig. 1.

The history of IOL implantation from the very beginning up to the highly sophisticated level we have achieved today is a very good example for progress. It took about 4000 years from the first documented description of cataract surgery in the Codex Hammurapi to the first successful IOL implantation in 1949 by Harold Ridley. After this first heroic IOL implantation, it was a long and hard way from monofocal PMMA IOLs, first implanted in the posterior chamber, after a detour to anterior chamber IOLs and pupil fixated IOLs, to the first foldable IOL implanted in the bag. Achievements such as phacoemulsification, viscoelastics, capsulorhexis, small incisions, limbal relaxing incisions and topical anesthesia were all implemented during that interesting time period. Especially astigmatism neutral surgery made the introduction of multifocal, toric and combined multifocal–toric, additive and extended range of vision IOLs possible. All these innovations were necessary

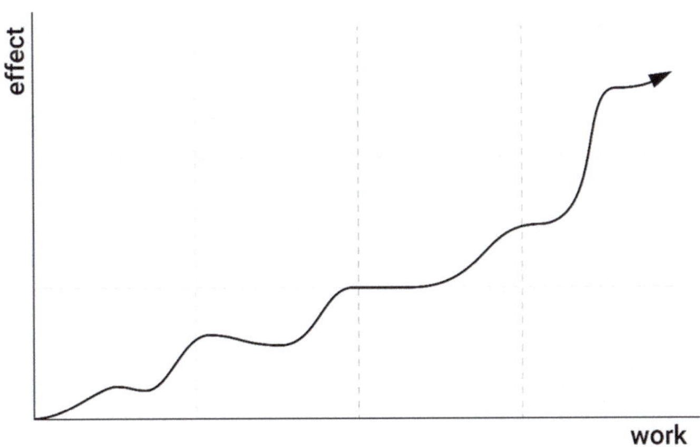

Fig. 1 Function of progress

to bring us to this high standard of patient care. Up until today, we have reached such a high surgical level that we do perform intraocular lens surgery not only in cataract cases but also for simple, refractive purposes. But even now we still need to implement a huge list of achievements in order to master the last frontier of IOL surgery, which is the perfect simulation of our physiological, juvenile lens, providing us with the full range of accommodation, full contrast and color perception.

One of the problems we as eye surgeons are confronted with more and more within the last decades is the incidence of late dislocation of the IOL/capsule complex. A lot of situations with incomplete capsular support or with aphakia prompt us to find creative surgical solutions for each specific case. No matter, if we have to deal with aphakic cases after pediatric cataract surgery, with cases after trauma or intraoperative capsule or zonular complications, with genetic diseases resulting in a lack of sufficient zonular support (e.g., Marfan syndrome, Marchesani syndrome), with PEX, high myopia, metabolic diseases or with the need of IOL exchange because of optic phenomena, mainly after multifocal IOL implantation or after any other cause, we need to find the best, stable and least traumatic solution in these situations.

With this book, we aim to highlight the great achievements made in order to overcome these challenging situations with different flanging techniques. Here again it was a typical curve of progress and each innovation, and each work helped to optimize surgery. As flanging techniques represent a very demanding surgery, one aim of this book is to steepen the learning curve and to encourage surgeons to add the presented techniques to their surgical armamentarium. We will describe the evolution of flanging surgery, the different approaches of flanging in anterior segment surgery, and we aim to give detailed background information in this evolving surgical field.

Liliana Werner, the world-known expert in the field of pathophysiology of IOLs, will present different causes of lens luxation in depth. She was one of the first authors who presented histological data on the "dead bag syndrome", one of the causes for late IOL dislocation.

Gabor Scharioth first described his great innovation of scleral tunnel fixation utilizing open-loop haptics, a technique that is widely accepted and performed. Even the gluing technique is based on that innovation. This technique was the basis of the next steps in our ascending wave of progress. He will describe the development of this technique from the very beginning.

Shin Yamane revolutionized scleral tunnel fixation with his brilliant idea of using a thin-walled 30G needle for haptic externalization and flanging the two haptic ends with cautery. He will describe his technique in detail and will show tricks for successful surgery.

Sergio Canabrava modified the option of flanging and described the elegant double-flange technique for sutures, a technique where closed-loop IOLs are fixed to the sclera by flanging both ends of a polypropylene suture. In his chapter, he will describe the history and evolution of this technique.

Ehud Assia, the inventor of different fixation devices for the capsular bag, will present exquisite techniques for the fixation of devices and IOLs with flanged sutures. He will also show his approach for fixation of IOLs by creating holes to IOL optics.

Even though it is impossible to describe and discuss the plethora of surgical techniques, implants and instruments completely, we will try to create a systematic approach for decision-making in a separate chapter. There are so many different cases to be treated and not all cases should be treated the same way. We have to decide if an IOL exchange is necessary or if we can refixate the IOL/capsule compartment, the latter being less traumatic in some situations. We also have to decide which fixation technique will work best in each patient.

Wolfgang Geitzenauer, Konstantin Seiller-Tarbuk and I will review the utilization of optimized instruments and implants. In this chapter, we will describe instruments facilitating flanging procedures, will discuss IOL selection for different purposes and present experimental data about flanging.

Finally, the authors will share surgical pearls and answer questions on the promising field of flanging surgery.

Surgical techniques with their specific details are ideally presented using videos. To get the most out of this book, all chapters include links to online videos from our own surgical cases.

As always when adopting disruptive ideas in our routine, we have to overcome difficulties. Every surgeon has to find surgical solutions he/she is comfortable with. As there exist so many different surgical techniques, instruments and implants, this book should help every surgeon to steepen the learning curve significantly, should give new inspiration and should help to find the best individual approach for the cure of our patients.

I am honored that all these outstanding innovators in the field accepted to contribute to the book about this hot topic.

Vienna, Austria   Michael Amon
                                                                           amon@augenchirurg.com

Acknowledgements

I want to thank my colleagues, authors and innovators Ehud Assia, Sergio Canabrava, Gabor Scharioth, Liliana Werner and Shin Yamane for the enormous contribution they gave within this book and for their disruptive work in ophthalmology. I also thank Wolfgang Geitzenauer, Konstantin Seiller-Tarbuk and all co-authors for their tremendous work within this project. I want to thank my mentor Heinz Freyler, who gave me great inspiration from the very beginning. I also want to thank my colleagues at my working place, who help me so much in our daily routine. Especially my mother Elfriede, my father Helmut, my sister Birgit, my brother Alexander, my daughter Daria, my son Michael Arian and my wife Martina brought love and motivation into my life. Without all these people, this book would not exist.

Vienna, Austria

Michael Amon
amon@augenchirurg.com

Contents

Causes of Intraocular Lens Dislocation 1
Liliana Werner

From Anterior Chamber IOLs to Scleral Tunnel Fixation of IOLs 15
Gabor B. Scharioth

Flanging 3-Piece IOLs 41
Shin Yamane

History and Evolution of Double Flanged Suture Fixation 49
Sérgio Canabrava

Flanging Intraocular Lenses and Devices in Special Situations 55
Avner Belkin and Ehud I. Assia

Decision-Making: IOL Refixation, IOL Exchange and Correction of Aphakia 67
Michael Amon, Wolfgang Geitzenauer, and Konstantin Seiller-Tarbuk

Utilizing Optimized Instruments and Implants 99
Wolfgang Geitzenauer, Konstantin Seiller-Tarbuk, and Michael Amon

Pearls from the Authors and Answers to Important Questions 119
Michael Amon

About the Editor

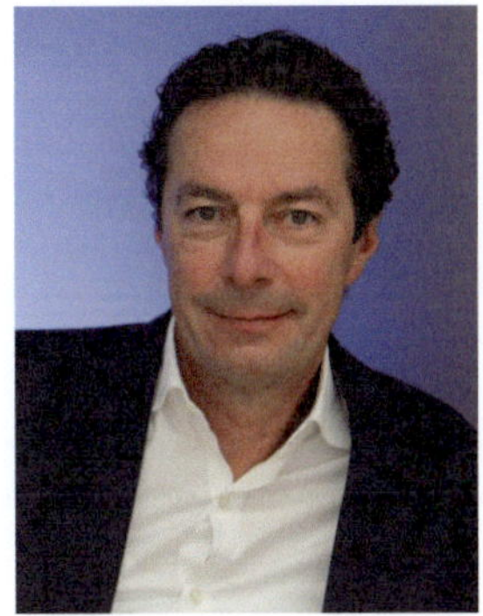

Michael Amon M.D. is the chairman of the Sigmund Freud Medical University and the head of the eye department at the Academic Teaching Hospital of St. John Vienna. In 2009, he was awarded a professorship by the Medical University Vienna. He was an Austrian delegate for EBO and UEMS, a board member and the congress president of DGII and the president of the Austrian and Viennese Ophthalmological Society. He was a board member of the ESCRS and is a board member of the Austrian Ophthalmological Society and the head of the Austrian Cataract Committee. Since 2012, he is a member of the Education Committee of the ESCRS. In a citation analysis in 2008, he was cited as the 5th influential author in Europe and 20th worldwide. He is the member of several editorial boards and of the IIIC. Besides different intraocular implants, he invented the first single-piece add-on IOL and different surgical instruments. With the development of the term "uveal and capsular biocompatibility", he underlined his main scientific interest in IOLs and in cataract surgery in compromised eyes. He has performed over 30,000 intraocular procedures, including pediatric cataract, posterior segment, glaucoma and corneal surgeries. He organized main symposia, instructional courses and wet laboratoriess, chaired sessions, presented on learning platforms and performed live surgery at international and national congresses.

Causes of Intraocular Lens Dislocation

Liliana Werner

Abstract

In this chapter, we examine risk factors for postoperative intraocular lens (IOL) dislocation, possible relationship with specific IOL materials and designs, as well as outcomes of cases with and without the use of a capsular tension ring (CTR).

Keywords

Intraocular lens · Dislocation · Pseudoexfoliation · Capsular tension ring · Dead bag syndrome

Introduction

Ectopia Lentis

Ectopia lentis is a term used to describe dislocation or displacement of the natural crystalline lens [1]. The crystalline lens is defined as luxated (dislocated) when it lies completely outside of the hyaloid fossa, is free-floating in the vitreous, is in the anterior chamber, or lies directly on the retina. The crystalline lens is considered subluxated when it is partially displaced but remains within the lens space. Ectopia lentis can occur due to trauma, as well as ocular or systemic diseases, usually representing genetic disorders. Ocular diseases associated with ectopia lentis include simple ectopia lentis, ectopia lentis et pupillae, aniridia, congenital glaucoma, pseudoexfoliation (PEX) syndrome,

L. Werner (✉)

Ophthalmology and Visual Sciences, Intermountain Ocular Research Center, John A. Moran Eye Center, University of Utah, 65 Mario Capecchi Drive, Salt Lake City, UT 84132, USA
e-mail: liliana.werner@hsc.utah.edu

M. Amon (ed.), *Flanging Techniques in Anterior Segment Surgery*,
https://doi.org/10.1007/978-3-031-32855-8_1

syphilis, retinitis pigmentosa, intraocular tumor, Axenfeld Rieger syndrome, mega-locornea, hypermature cataract, high myopia, buphthalmos, as well as anterior uveal tumors. Systemic diseases associated with ectopia lentis include Marfan syndrome, homocystinuria, Weill-Marchesani syndrome, sulfite oxidase deficiency, hyperlysinemia, Ehlers-Danlos syndrome, Sturge-Weber syndrome, mandibulofacial dysostosis, Wildervanck syndrome, Conradi syndrome, Pfaundler syndrome, Crouzon syndrome, Pierre Robin syndrome, as well as Sprengel deformity.

Surgical management of ectopia lentis is usually indicated when there is progressive lens subluxation, cataract formation, lens instability, pupil block glaucoma, or retinal detachment [2]. While preservation of the capsular bag with in-the-bag intraocular lens (IOL) implantation, usually in association with implantation of a capsular device for scleral fixation (e.g., modified capsular tension ring—CTR), may be possible in cases of subluxated crystalline lenses with limited zonular support, management with lensectomy/vitrectomy will require an alternative form of IOL fixation, when an IOL is used for the correction of aphakia.

Intraocular Lens Dislocation

The focus of this chapter is, however, on the causes of postoperative dislocation of artificial IOLs used in cataract surgery. IOLs appear to dislocate in a bimodal distribution [3, 4]. Early IOL dislocation is generally defined as occurring less than 3 months postoperatively. It is usually secondary to poor IOL fixation; therefore, its rate has decreased since the advent of continuous curvilinear capsulorrhexis (CCC). The incidence of posterior chamber IOL decentration/dislocation after complicated cataract surgery ranges between 0.2 and 3.0%, usually manifesting in the first weeks after surgery [5].

Late postoperative IOL dislocation is defined as occurring 3 months or more after surgery. In-the-bag dislocation occurs as a result of progressive zonular dehiscence after even uneventful surgery, not from inadequate IOL fixation. This complication is described to occur as a continuum from pseudophacodonesis, through subluxation, to dislocation of the IOL–capsule complex into the vitreous cavity or the anterior chamber (total dislocation) [5]. Some patients have acute vision loss, whereas others experience more subtle symptoms, such as glare, halos, diplopia, or oscillating vision over a longer period of time, as well as gradual visual impairment, depending on the degree of dislocation. Late in-the-bag IOL dislocation occurs on average 6–12 years after cataract surgery, and the mean patient age varies between 65 and 85 years [5].

Major risk factors for zonulysis and late in-the-bag dislocation include trauma and conditions leading to progressive zonular weakness. This later is a well-described feature in eyes with PEX syndrome (considered the most common risk factor), high myopia, uveitis, as well as certain connective tissue disorders including Marfan's syndrome, homocystinuria, hyperlysinemia, Ehlers-Danlos syndrome, scleroderma, and Weil-Marchesani's syndrome. Zonular weakness may be observed after vitreoretinal surgery; zonules also become more friable as patients age, especially in PEX patients [6]. In a study examining the frequency of IOL dislocation and pseudophacodonesis 20 years after cataract surgery, the cumulative incidence over 20 years was 6% in patients with PEX and 2% in patients without PEX at surgery [7].

Trends for late in-the-bag IOL dislocations have been specifically investigated in a cohort study from Sweden, which found that the incidence of late in-the-bag IOL dislocation increased over a 20-year period, even after adjusting for the growing pseudophakic population [8]. Hypotheses proposed to explain this finding included a longer mean duration of pseudophakia in the population (years at risk) and potentially a lower threshold in recent years for performing phacoemulsification cataract surgery on more challenging cases that have a higher risk for dislocation [5].

Late In-the-Bag Intraocular Lens Dislocation and Pseudoexfoliation

Zonular Apparatus

The zonules are anchored by integrating in a mat-like fashion within the intrinsic fibers of the anterior and posterior capsules, approximately 2 mm anterior or posterior to the equator. A small subset of zonules inserts into the equator of the lens capsule, but they seem to bear a much smaller force load. The anterior and posterior zonules radiate centripetally in a coronal plane and intermix within the valleys of the pars plicata, forming a complicated plexus. Some of the fibers from the plexus attach to the valley walls of the pars plicata, stabilizing the plexus to the pars plicata. After attaching to the pars plicata, the zonules change direction and radiate posteriorly along the pars plana until they insert within the pars plana again intermingling in a mat-like fashion with the intrinsic fibers of the ciliary epithelial basement membrane. Zonular disruption anywhere along the course could cause zonular insufficiency [9].

Pseudoexfoliation

PEX is a condition in which abnormal extracellular matrix and basement membrane structural and metabolic proteins are deposited into virtually all structures within the anterior chamber. The PEX material is composed of a fibrillin and glycoprotein skeleton surrounded by an amorphous matrix of associated proteins. Lens epithelial cells (LECs) and ciliary epithelial cells deposit PEX material within their respective basement membrane lamellae. PEX accumulations mechanically weaken the zonular lamella and impair zonular anchoring to the epithelial basement membrane at both its origin and insertion. Because zonules mainly are composed of elastic fibers and patients with PEX exhibit an increase in elastinolysis, the disease likely also enzymatically weakens the zonules. Zonular disarticulation from the anchoring points at the basement membranes of the pars plicata, pars plana, or lens capsule initially produces phacodonesis and finally, when enough zonules are breached, lens capsule dislocation and displacement [10].

PEX is frequently associated with capsular contraction syndrome [11]. Capsular fibrosis promoting capsulorrhexis phimosis is another mechanism leading to zonular weakness. The phimosis exerts a tractional force on the capsular bag that is transmitted to the zonules. Capsular contraction syndrome may lead to zonulysis by itself; however, any capsular fibrosis may transmit increased force into the zonular apparatus. This force is not likely to be absorbed symmetrically by the zonules [10].

Pathological Studies Performed in Our Laboratory: Late In-the-Bag Intraocular Lens Dislocation and Pseudoexfoliation

Complete histopathologic analysis of selected specimens represented by capsular bags containing an IOL or an IOL and a CTR sometimes showed the presence of PEX material, even if there were no clinical history or evidence of PEX [12, 13]. We hypothesized that the prevalence of PEX might be higher in late postoperative in-the-bag IOL dislocation than the rate reported based on the clinical diagnosis of this condition. Therefore, we performed a study involving complete histopathologic analysis of a large series of capsular bags from such cases, consecutively explanted in the same center in Germany [14]. The specimens were represented by 40 capsular bags containing an IOL (N = 37) or an IOL–CTR (N = 3). Twenty-six specimens had histopathologic evidence of PEX, while only 13 had a clinical history or clinical evidence of PEX (including 2 cases with a CTR).

In the specimens with PEX (Fig. 1), the mean age at explantation was 80.5 ± 6.8 years with a mean time of 11.9 ± 5.2 years between implantation and explantation. These specimens came from 17 women and 9 men. Associated conditions according to the submitted questionnaires included glaucoma (N = 4), history of vitrectomy (N = 3), myopia (N = 1), retinal detachment (N = 1), and endophthalmitis (N = 1). The explanted IOLs included 10 three-piece hydrophobic acrylic lenses, 6 single-piece hydrophobic acrylic lenses, 4 three-piece silicone lenses, 3 single-piece hydrophilic acrylic lenses, 2 three-piece hydrophilic acrylic lenses, and 1 single-piece PMMA lens. Proliferative material within the capsular bags (Soemmering's ring formation) was present in all specimens, and was graded as mild in 3 specimens, moderate in 13 specimens, and severe in 10 specimens. LECs were also present in all specimens in some degree, but there were abundant LECs in 16 of the capsules and multiple layers of LECs in an additional 4 capsules. Capsular phimosis was also present in 17 of the 26 specimens [14].

For the 14 specimens without evidence of PEX (Fig. 2), the mean age at explantation was 71.8 ± 11.9 years, and there was a mean time of 12.2 ± 4.2 years between implantation and explantation. The specimens were from 9 women and 5 men, and the associated conditions according to the submitted questionnaires

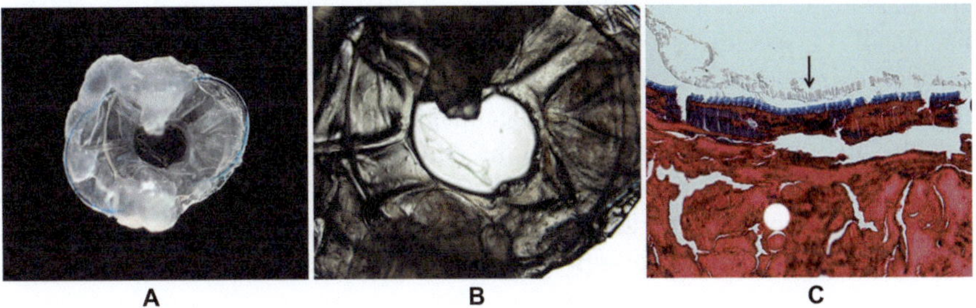

Fig. 1 Gross, light microscopic, and histopathologic photographs of an explanted three-piece hydrophobic acrylic IOL–capsular bag complex. A: Gross photograph of the IOL–capsular bag complex showing capsulorhexis phimosis and moderate Soemmering's ring formation. B: Light microscopic photograph of the IOL–capsular bag complex showing prominent anterior capsule folds (original magnification ×40). C: Histopathologic photograph of a section cut through the center of the IOL–capsular bag complex (Masson's trichrome stain) showing a continuous layer of PEX material on the anterior surface of the anterior capsule (arrow) (original magnification ×200). From: Liu E, Cole S, Werner L, Hengerer F, Mamalis N, Kohnen T (2015) Pathologic evidence of pseudoexfoliation in cases of in-the-bag intraocular lens subluxation or dislocation. J Cataract Refract Surg 41:929–935

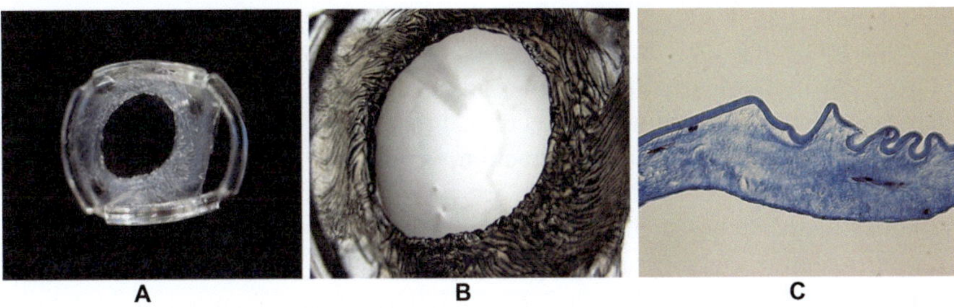

Fig. 2 Gross, light microscopic, and histopathologic photographs of an explanted single-piece hydrophilic acrylic IOL–capsular bag complex. A: Gross photograph of the IOL–capsular bag complex showing severe capsulorhexis phimosis and anterior flexing of the IOL haptics. B: Light microscopic photograph of the IOL–capsular bag complex showing prominent anterior capsule folds (original magnification ×40). C: Histopathologic photograph of a section cut through the center of the IOL–capsular bag complex (Masson's trichrome stain). Although there is dense anterior subcapsular fibrosis and fibrous metaplasia of the anterior LECs, no histopathologic evidence of PEX material is present (original magnification ×400). From: Liu E, Cole S, Werner L, Hengerer F, Mamalis N, Kohnen T (2015) Pathologic evidence of pseudoexfoliation in cases of in-the-bag intraocular lens subluxation or dislocation. J Cataract Refract Surg 41:929–935

were myopia (N = 3), history of vitrectomy (N = 2), retinal detachment (N = 1), zonular loss (N = 1), retinitis pigmentosa (N = 1), Marfan syndrome (N = 1), and history of trauma (N = 1). The explanted IOLs included 3 three-piece hydrophobic acrylic lenses, 1 single-piece hydrophobic acrylic lens, 2 three-piece silicone lenses, 3 single-piece hydrophilic acrylic lenses, and 5 single-piece PMMA lenses.

Histopathologic examination of the specimens showed Soemmering's ring formation in all 14 specimens (mild N = 5, moderate N = 5, severe N = 4) and capsulorhexis phimosis in 7 specimens. LECs were also present in all 14 specimens but only abundant in 3 of the specimens. In that study [14], our hypothesis that PEX may be more prevalent than the rate based on clinical assessment alone was confirmed, and it is possible that ultrastructural evaluations (e.g., transmission electron microscopy) would have yielded an even higher PEX rate than that found based on histopathologic analyses.

Late In-the-Bag Intraocular Lens Dislocation With and Without a Capsular Tension Ring

Pathological Studies Performed in Our Laboratory: Late In-the-Bag Intraocular Lens Dislocation Without a Capsular Tension Ring

In a 2021 review paper on late in-the-bag IOL dislocation, the authors reported that some of the studies included in the review have indicated a possible association between dislocation of the IOL-capsular bag complex and certain IOL designs and materials [5]. However, the results were inconsistent, and when associations were found, they likely reflected the IOL types most frequently used in the years preceding the corresponding studies. In analyses of pseudophakic eyes obtained postmortem [15, 16], as well as clinical studies [17], plate–haptic silicone IOLs have been associated with an increased risk for anterior capsule opacification (ACO) with secondary capsule contraction, which may subsequently increase the risk for dislocation. In our laboratory, we performed pathological studies on late in-the-bag dislocations, including specimens with [12] and without a CTR [13].

A retrospective study included explanted IOLs within the capsular bag evaluated from March 2000 through March 2008 [12]. They were submitted to the laboratory immersed in fixative, such as 10% neutral buffered formalin. The specimens were analyzed macro and microscopically for IOL design, IOL material composition, and any notable pathologic features. Surgeons were also asked to submit a case summary with the specimen by answering a questionnaire regarding the patient's age, gender, history leading to dislocation, cause requiring IOL explantation, exchange IOL design, and dates of IOL implantation and explantation. Chart review, where obtainable, confirmed the survey data.

Eighty-six IOLs that were dislocated within the capsular bag were obtained over this 8-year period. Fifty-nine of the total 86 IOLs were submitted from January 2006 through March 2008. This series included polymethylmethacrylate (PMMA; N = 28), silicone (N = 33), and hydrophobic acrylic (N = 25) lenses that were single-piece or three-piece designs. Hydrophilic acrylic lenses were not represented, likely because all specimens came from surgeons within the USA, and these lenses were not popular in the USA at that time. Of the available data, 43 IOLs were explanted from males and 37 were explanted from females. The mean age of the patients at explantation was 75 years (±13 years), and patient age ranged from 31 to 93 years. Identified associated conditions included PEX, previous vitreoretinal surgery, previous history of trauma, and uveitis. Excluding 1 outlying patient who underwent implantation more than 25 years before explantation, the mean time from implantation to explantation was 8.5 years (range, 3 months–17 years). Thirty-six percent of capsular bags contained no cortical material, whereas 30% contained a minimal amount of material, 27% contained a moderate amount of material, and 7% contained a large or severe amount of cortical material. Of those that contained a large or severe amount of cortical material, 3 cases were associated with PEX and 1 with uveitis. Capsular fibrosis was found to be a significant finding from the specimens, and cases of typical capsular contraction syndrome were observed with all IOL materials and designs [12].

IOL dislocation was associated with PEX in 15 males and 24 females. The mean age of patients with PEX and dislocated IOLs was 81 years (±7.5 years), a statistically significant (P = 0.02, Student t test) 6 years older than the mean population dislocation age (75 years). Ages at dislocation ranged from 62 to 93 years. The mean time from lens implantation to explantation was 8.4 years (±3.1 years). Explantation time ranged from 4 to 17 years after surgery. There were 18 cases of capsular contraction syndrome in the PEX group, 3 involving single-piece PMMA lenses, 4 plate-haptic silicone lenses, 6 three-piece hydrophobic acrylic lenses, 3 three-piece silicone lenses, and 4 single-piece hydrophobic acrylic lenses with haptics [12].

There were 13 male patients and 3 female patients with dislocation associated with vitreoretinal surgery. The mean age of the patients was 68 years (±9.4 years), a statistically significant (P = 0.02, Student t test) 7 years younger than the population mean age at dislocation. The mean length of time from implantation to explantation was 10 years (range, 1 month–25 years). The mean time corrected to exclude the outlier with a more than 25-year gap from implantation to explantation was 8.5 years. There were 5 cases of capsular contraction syndrome in this group, 1 involving a plate-haptic silicone lens, 2 involving three-piece silicone lenses, and 2 involving single-piece hydrophobic acrylic lenses with haptics [12]. Little scientific literature exists that discusses the effect of pars plana vitrectomy on the zonular apparatus. Introduction of trocars through the overlying sclera and pars plana likely traumatizes zonules at their insertion. Port manipulation throughout the vitreoretinal procedure likely continues the mechanical trauma initiated by the introduction of trocars. Because of the geometry of the zonular apparatus, focal surgical disruption of zonules unevenly distributes the increases in stress on the remaining intact zonules. Other factors like vitrector energy delivered indirectly to the zonules, intraoperative and postoperative pressure changes within the globe, and postoperative inflammation also may contribute to the zonular insufficiency [18].

Capsular Tension Ring

In the above-mentioned study, none of the specimens contained an accompanying CTR, which indirectly suggested the efficacy of this device in preventing late in-the-bag IOL dislocation [12]. The CTR is used as an intraoperative support tool during cataract surgery, and as a long-term implant device for postoperative IOL fixation. It acts by expanding the capsular bag, and recruiting and redistributing tension from existing zonules, which leads to reinforcement of areas of weak zonules, and recentration of a mildly subluxated capsular bag. Standard CTRs are usually indicated in cases of mild zonular instability, with zonulysis observed in less than 3 to 4 clock-hours, or signs of mild degree of zonular weakness such as mild phacodonesis. Common indications include PEX, traumatic or iatrogenic zonular damage, Marfan syndrome, homocystinuria, hypermature cataracts, and post vitrectomy and filtration patients [19, 20]. A study using human eyes obtained postmortem showed that, in terms of minimizing further zonular stress and damage and capsular destabilization, the ideal timing for CTR placement is after lens extraction and decompression of the capsular bag [21]. There is, however, debate as to the optimal timing of CTR in-the-bag insertion [22].

Pathological Studies Performed in Our Laboratory: Late In-the-Bag Intraocular Lens Dislocation with a Capsular Tension Ring

In a follow-up pathological study, 23 specimens corresponding to explanted subluxated or dislocated capsular bags containing a CTR and an IOL were evaluated [13]. Explantation was performed a mean of 81.5 ± 32.2 months after implantation (approximately 6.8 years). Available information on associated ocular conditions included PEX (74%), glaucoma (17%), vitrectomy or retina surgery (13%), and trauma (4%). Excessive contraction of the capsular bag with capsulorhexis phimosis was observed in 11 specimens, 1 with an associated history of vitrectomy, 7 with an associated history of PEX, and 3 with an associated history of glaucoma. One of the eyes had implantation of a single-piece hydrophilic acrylic IOL; excessive capsule fibrosis led to capsulorhexis phimosis and anterior flexing of the IOL haptics despite the presence of a CTR (Fig. 3). Explantation was performed a mean of 72.1 ± 41.3 months after implantation (approximately 6 years) in eyes with capsulorhexis phimosis.

It is not surprising that the mean explantation time was shorter in the series of 23 specimens containing a CTR (6.8 or 6.0 years, without or with capsulorhexis phimosis, respectively) [13] than in the series of 86 specimens without a CTR (8.5 years) [12], considering that CTRs are usually implanted when zonular weakness is already observed before or during surgery. This has also been reported in other series by different authors [23]. Stress to the zonular fibers during CTR insertion cannot be ruled out [21].

The question has been raised as to whether CTRs should be used prophylactically in a patient with a history of PEX or vitreoretinal surgery with no phacodonesis at the time of cataract surgery. This is a reasonable question considering not just the apparent increasing number of spontaneously dislocated lenses [8], but also the many dislocated lenses that may be repositioned and fixated to the iris or sclera without explantation [24]. When weighing the added cost and time to

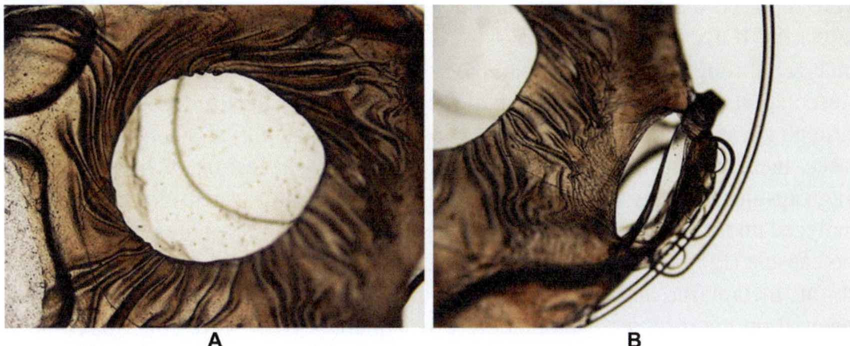

Fig. 3 Light microscopic photographs of an explanted single-piece hydrophilic acrylic IOL–capsular bag complex also containing a CTR showing fibrous metaplasia, contraction of the capsular bag, and capsulorhexis phimosis with multiple anterior capsular folds (A), as well as anterior flexing of the closed loops of the lens (B)

perform the procedure with the relatively low incidence of dislocation within the general population, generalized, prophylactic use does not appear advisable. However, in a study using the documentation database of 1 hospital, cataract surgeries and in-the-bag IOL dislocations were evaluated over a period of 21 years to determine the role of a CTR implantation in the development of this complication and assessment of risk factors. A subgroup analysis of a CTR implantation in eyes with and without PEX showed a significantly reduced risk of in-the-bag IOL dislocation if a CTR was used in eyes with PEX, which was not the case in eyes without PEX [25]. Certainly, CTRs are indicated with any sign of zonular insufficiency; however, even if there is a reduced risk, its presence does not necessarily prevent late in-the-bag IOL dislocation. In case this complication occurs, repositioning can be performed by using different surgical techniques specifically described taking into account the presence of this device in the capsular bag [26, 27].

Late In-the-Bag Intraocular Lens Dislocation and Dead Bag Syndrome

Since the early 2000s, there have been presentations and discussions at different meetings and online forums about IOL dislocation cases where the capsular bag itself had apparently become diaphanous and floppy, and unable to support the IOL within it. The common feature among those cases appeared to be the presence of a very clear capsular bag many years after surgery. Sam Masket from Los Angeles, CA, USA was the first to observe the condition and coined the term "dead bag syndrome" to refer to them. The first peer-reviewed study on this syndrome, to the best of my knowledge, was published by our group in February 2022 [28]. Ten cases were included in that article, with a mean time between implantation and explantation (when performed) of 10.6 ± 5.6 years. No signs of zonular instability were reported during the implantation surgeries, which were all uneventful. In 7 cases, the IOLs and capsular bags were explanted, and all 7 capsular bags were analyzed through detailed histopathology, as well as 5 of the 7 explanted IOLs. At presentation, there was subluxation of the IOL inside of the floppy bag, sometimes through a peripheral defect, while the capsular bag itself was still centered. In other cases, there was in-the-bag IOL dislocation. The main feature of histopathology was capsular splitting or delamination. LECs were rarely seen in the specimens analyzed under histopathology, or were completely absent from the inner surface of the capsule (Fig. 4). Only one capsular bag specimen had mild amounts of anterior fibrous metaplasia, and another capsular bag contained a small amount of cortical material on microscopic examination. The explanted IOLs were either three-piece silicone, or single-piece hydrophobic acrylic IOLs, and were unremarkable under light microscopy aside from mild pigmentary dispersion on their surfaces [28].

Three other cases of possible dead bag syndrome were also included in the same study. In one of them, only the IOL was explanted; inferior dislocation of the single-piece IOL into the vitreous cavity occurred through a peripheral/posterior capsular defect, while the residual capsular bag still appeared to have appropriate zonular support. In this case, sulcus fixation of a three-piece hydrophobic acrylic lens with posterior optic capture was done. In the other two cases, explantation of the IOL or the capsular bag was not found necessary although, in one of them, nasal zonulysis has been observed more recently [28].

Histopathological findings of the dead bag syndrome capsules were compared to those of capsules from 40 cases of in-the-bag IOL dislocation, including 26 cases with evident pseudoexfoliation material [14]. LECs and Soemmering's ring

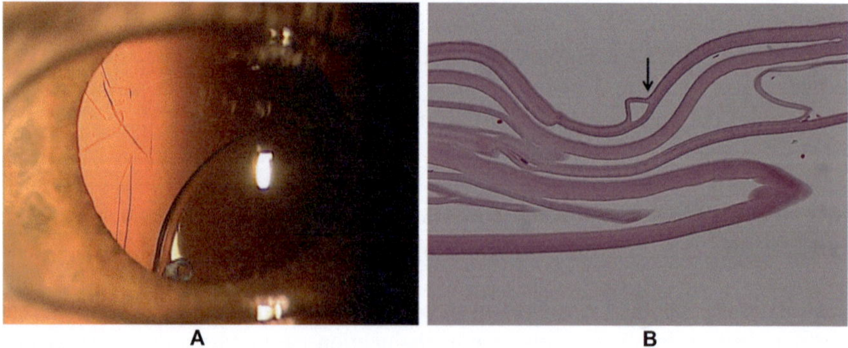

A   B

Fig. 4 Dead Bag Syndrome. A: Slitlamp photograph of a suspected dead bag syndrome case, showing IOL subluxation and a remarkably clear capsule. B: Light photomicrograph of a histopathological section cut from the capsular bag in A, showing a site of capsular splitting (arrow), and almost no LECs attached to the capsule (hematoxylin–eosin stain, original magnification ×200). From: Culp C, Qu P, Jones J, Fram N, Ogawa G, Masket S, Mamalis N, Werner L (2022) Clinical and histopathological findings in the dead bag syndrome. J Cataract Refract Surg 48:177–184

formation were observed in all cases; capsulorhexis phimosis was also a relatively common finding, while capsular splitting/delamination was only found in 1 specimen. A review of the literature indicates there is also capsular splitting/delamination in true exfoliation syndrome [29]. However, in this condition, which may be associated with chronic exposure to intense heat or infrared radiation, there is usually a thin membrane of delaminated capsule on the anterior surface of the crystalline lens before cataract surgery. Specific differences with the above-mentioned conditions show dead bag syndrome to be a distinct entity.

The exact etiology of dead bag syndrome is still unknown. We hypothesize that late postoperative zonular failure is related to capsule splitting/delamination occurring at the level of zonular attachments. This syndrome does not appear to have any association with a particular IOL design or material. When looking at the results of our first peer-reviewed study on this syndrome, especially regarding the scarcity of LECs in the capsules, many surgeons are naturally asking the question whether capsular polishing has any relationship with this syndrome. However, no clear association between polishing and dead bag syndrome could be established so far. Cortical lens fibers and LECs continue to deposit extracellular matrix and lens capsule components at their basal ends, which contributes to the thickening of the capsule throughout life, as well as maintaining its integrity [30]. There has been a recent emphasis on polishing techniques to prevent capsular bag opacification, especially in association with premium lenses [31–34]. Nevertheless, even extensive polishing cannot completely remove all LECs. Furthermore, polishing is usually not done at the capsular bag equator, as this region is not readily visible. Masket has also observed cases of white, intumescent cataracts that evolved into dead bag syndrome, suggesting that there may be a role of oncotic pressure within the capsular bag in killing LECs. However, many dead bag cases are not related to this type of cataract, and other factors are likely involved in its origin.

Discussions on the dead bag syndrome done in online forums described many apparent dead bag cases that were not associated with extensive polishing, as well as cases where the capsule was floppy and delicate, but still exhibited a certain amount of proliferative material within it, including abnormal gel-like Soemmering's ring formation. It is possible that the findings described in our first publication may represent the severe end of a spectrum [28]. The relationship between LECs and the capsule, especially post cataract surgery is not yet fully understood. While as noted above, LECs are important for the formation of the capsule, this structure represents an anchor point for the basal surfaces of epithelial and fiber cells, also providing necessary signals for proper lens cell proliferation, migration and differentiation [35]. Another possibility in the dead bag syndrome is that the initial problem is in the capsule itself, which would initiate a cycle of LEC damage with further damage to the capsule. There are many unanswered questions not only about the etiology of this syndrome, but also in its manifestations. Management is therefore currently advised on a case-by-case basis, depending on presentation, as well as status of the zonular support.

Conclusions

Early postoperative IOL dislocation is usually secondary to poor IOL fixation, while late postoperative IOL dislocation is usually a result of zonular weakness. Major risk factors for zonulysis and late in-the-bag IOL dislocation include trauma and conditions leading to progressive zonular weakness, especially PEX. Late in-the-bag IOL dislocation may occur after implantation of any type of IOL, and the amount of proliferative/regenerative material within the capsular bag in dislocated specimens appears to vary largely. Excessive fibrosis of the bag is a frequent finding. The cumulative incidence of this complication appears to be increasing with time, and surgeons must be prepared to eventually deal with it. Management depends on surgeon's preferences and specialty, type of IOL implanted, presence or not of a CTR, stage and site of dislocation, as well as coexisting ocular pathology. Surgical approaches include different methods for repositioning, or for exchange. Different conditions leading to zonular weakness, such as PEX are progressive, and although standard CTRs can provide initial support, they do not appear to completely prevent capsulorhexis phimosis or late dislocation. In cases of more profound zonular weakness, devices designed for scleral fixation should be considered, as there is a fine line between zonular insufficiency that can be stabilized with the standard CTR alone and that requiring further support.

It is important to keep in mind that PEX can be a difficult clinical diagnosis, with many cases going unnoticed until well advanced. This condition is likely present in a much larger percentage of patients who had late in-the-bag IOL dislocation than the number currently detected clinically. The dead bag syndrome is another condition that has been increasingly recognized as leading to late IOL subluxation/dislocation. Contrary to PEX, in which abnormal extracellular matrix and basement membrane structural and metabolic proteins are deposited into virtually all structures within the anterior chamber, mechanically weaken the zonular lamella, in the dead bag syndrome, late postoperative zonular failure appears to be related to capsule splitting/delamination occurring at the level of zonular attachments. This condition requires further studies.

References

1. Patel AS, Ringeisen AL, DelMonte DW, Hossain K, Morkin M, Puente MA, Gurnani B. Ectopia lentis. American Academy of Ophthalmology EyeWiki. 2015. https://eyewiki.aao.org/Ectopia_Lentis. Accessed 01 Dec 2022.
2. Chandra A, Charteris D. Molecular pathogenesis and management strategies of ectopia lentis. Eye (Lond). 2014;28:162–8.
3. Gimbel HV, Condon GP, Kohnen T, Olson RJ, Halkiadakis I. Late in-the-bag intraocular lens dislocation: incidence, prevention, and management. J Cataract Refract Surg. 2005;31:2193–204.
4. Hayashi K, Hirata A, Hayashi H. Possible predisposing factors for in-the-bag and out-of-the-bag intraocular lens dislocation and outcomes of intraocular lens exchange surgery. Ophthalmology. 2007;114:969–75.

5. Kristianslund O, Dalby M, Drolsum L. Late in-the-bag intraocular lens dislocation. J Cataract Refract Surg. 2021;47:942–54.

6. Mönestam EI. Incidence of dislocation of intraocular lenses and pseudophakodonesis 10 years after cataract surgery. Ophthalmology. 2009;116:2315–20.

7. Mönestam EI. Frequency of intraocular lens dislocation and pseudophacodonesis, 20 years after cataract surgery—a prospective study. Am J Ophthalmol. 2019;198:215–22.

8. Dabrowska-Kloda K, Kloda T, Boudiaf S, Jakobsson G, Stenevi U. Incidence and risk factors of late in-the-bag intraocular lens dislocation: evaluation of 140 eyes between 1992 and 2012. J Cataract Refract Surg. 2015;41:1376–82.

9. Rohen JW. Scanning electron microscopic studies of the zonular apparatus in human and monkey eyes. Invest Ophthalmol Vis Sci. 1979;18:133–44.

10. Schlötzer-Schrehardt U, Naumann GOH. Ocular and systemic pseudoexfoliation syndrome. Review Am J Ophthalmol. 2006;141:921–37.

11. Davison JA. Capsule contraction syndrome. J Cataract Refract Surg. 1993;19:582–9.

12. Davis D, Brubaker J, Espandar L, Stringham J, Crandall A, Werner L, Mamalis N. Late in-the-bag spontaneous intraocular lens dislocation: evaluation of 86 consecutive cases. Ophthalmology. 2009;116:664–70.

13. Werner L, Zaugg B, Neuhann T, Burrow M, Tetz M. In-the-bag capsular tension ring and intraocular lens subluxation or dislocation: a series of 23 cases. Ophthalmology. 2012;119:266–71.

14. Liu E, Cole S, Werner L, Hengerer F, Mamalis N, Kohnen T. Pathologic evidence of pseudoexfoliation in cases of in-the-bag intraocular lens subluxation or dislocation. J Cataract Refract Surg. 2015;41:929–35.

15. Werner L, Pandey SK, Escobar-Gomez M, Visessook N, Peng Q, Apple DJ. Anterior capsule opacification: a histopathological study comparing different IOL styles. Ophthalmology. 2000;107:463–71.

16. Werner L, Pandey SK, Apple DJ, Escobar-Gomez M, McLendon L, Macky TA. Anterior capsule opacification: correlation of pathologic findings with clinical sequelae. Ophthalmology. 2001;108:1675–81.

17. Hayashi K, Hayashi H, Nakao F, Hayashi F. Reduction in the area of the anterior capsule opening after polymethylmethacrylate, silicone, and soft acrylic intraocular lens implantation. Am J Ophthalmol. 1997;123:441–7.

18. Matsumoto M, Yamada K, Uematsu M, Fujikawa A, Tsuiki E, Kumagami T, Suzuma K, Kitaoka T. Spontaneous dislocation of in-the-bag intraocular lens primarily in cases with prior vitrectomy. Eur J Ophthalmol. 2012;22:363–7.

19. Menapace R, Findl O, Georgopoulos M, Rainer G, Vass C, Schmetterer K. The capsular tension ring: designs, applications, and techniques. J Cataract Refract Surg. 2000;26:898–912.

20. Hasanee K, Butler M, Ahmed II. Capsular tension rings and related devices: current concepts. Curr Opin Ophthalmol. 2006;17:31–41.

21. Ahmed II, Cionni RJ, Kranemann C, Crandall AS. Optimal timing of capsular tension ring implantation: Miyake-Apple video analysis. J Cataract Refract Surg. 2005;31:1809–13.

22. Fine IH, Hoffman RS, Packer M. Timing of CTR implantation. J Cataract Refract Surg. 2006;32(7):1075.

23. Lorente R, de Rojas V, Vazquez de Parga P, Moreno C, Landaluce ML, Domínguez R, Lorente B. Management of late spontaneous in-the-bag intraocular lens dislocation: retrospective analysis of 45 cases. J Cataract Refract Surg. 2010;36:1270–82.

24. Moreno-Montañés J, Rodriguez-Conde R. Capsular tension ring in eyes with pseudoexfoliation. J Cataract Refract Surg. 2002;28:2241–2.

25. Mayer-Xanthaki CF, Hirnschall N, Pregartner G, Gabriel M, Falb T, Sommer M, Haas A. Capsular tension ring as a protective measure against in-the-bag dislocations after cataract surgery. J Cataract Refract Surg. 2022. Online ahead of print.

26. Moreno-Montañés J, Heras H, Fernández-Hortelano A. Surgical treatment of a dislocated intraocular lens-capsular bag-capsular tension ring complex. J Cataract Refract Surg. 2005;31:270–3.

27. Ahmed II, Chen SH, Kranemann C, Wong DT. Surgical repositioning of dislocated capsular tension rings. Ophthalmology. 2005;112:1725–33.
28. Culp C, Qu P, Jones J, Fram N, Ogawa G, Masket S, Mamalis N, Werner L. Clinical and histopathological findings in the dead bag syndrome. J Cataract Refract Surg. 2022;48:177–84.
29. Cooke CA, Lum DJ, Wheeldon CE, Teoh H, McGhee CN. Surgical approach, histopathology, and pathogenesis in cataract associated with true lens exfoliation. J Cataract Refract Surg. 2007;33:735–8.
30. Danysh BP, Duncan MK. The lens capsule. Exp Eye Res. 2009;88:151–64.
31. Wang SB, Quah XM, Amjadi S, Tong J, Francis IC. Hydropolish: a controlled trial on a technique to eradicate residual cortical lens fibers in phacoemulsification cataract surgery. Eur J Ophthalmol. 2015;25:571–4.
32. Liu Z, Cao Q, Qu B, Wang W, Ruan X, Zheng D, Jin G, Tan X, Jin L, He M, Congdon N, Lin H, Luo L, Liu Y. Fluid-jet technique to polish the posterior capsule for phacoemulsification surgeries: efficacy and safety evaluation. J Cataract Refract Surg. 2020;46:1508–14.
33. Luft N, Kreutzer TC, Dirisamer M, Priglinger CS, Burger J, Findl O, Priglinger SG. Evaluation of laser capsule polishing for prevention of posterior capsule opacification in a human ex vivo model. J Cataract Refract Surg. 2015;41:2739–45.
34. Menapace R, Di Nardo S. Aspiration curette for anterior capsule polishing: laboratory and clinical evaluation. J Cataract Refract Surg. 2006;32:1997–2003.
35. Oharazawa H, Ibaraki N, Lin LR, Reddy VN. The effects of extracellular matrix on cell attachment, proliferation and migration in a human lens epithelial cell line. Exp Eye Res. 1999;69:603–10.

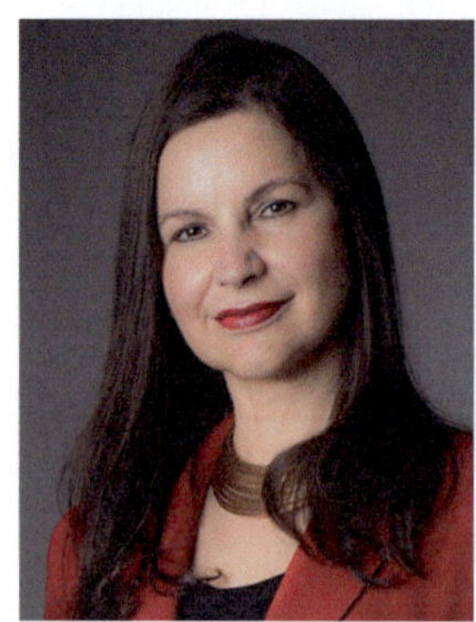

Liliana Werner, MD PhD is a Professor of Ophthalmology and Vision Sciences, and Co-Director of the Intermountain Ocular Research Center, at the John A. Moran Eye Center, University of Utah. She has a MD degree from Brazil, and a PhD degree (Biomaterials) from France. Dr. Werner's research is centered on the interaction between ocular tissues and different intraocular lens designs, materials and surface modifications. These include intraocular lenses implanted after cataract surgery, and also phakic lenses for refractive surgery and ophthalmic implantable devices in general. She has authored more than 360 peer-reviewed publications and book chapters on the subject, co-edited 3 books, and received numerous awards in international meetings for scientific presentations, videos and posters. She has also been a guest speaker in different international meetings in at least 25 countries, and a consultant for different companies manufacturing IOLs and other ocular biodevices. Since June 1st, 2020, Dr. Werner is the US Associate Editor of the Journal of Cataract & Refractive Surgery.

From Anterior Chamber IOLs to Scleral Tunnel Fixation of IOLs

Gabor B. Scharioth

Abstract

We will describe in detail technique for secondary implantation of PCIOL with intrascleral haptic fixation and its evolution and modifications. Focus is made on the description and illustration of each step of the Scharioth technique. Some variations including Glued IOL, implantation of multifocal IOL, single piece IOL and combined IOL and artificial iris are shown in this chapter.

Keywords

Intrascleral fixation · Scharioth technique · Glued IOL · Aphakia · Luxated IOL · Secondary implantation

An ophthalmic surgeon could be faced with three main scenarios. The patient could be aphakic after complicated phacoemulsification, trauma, vitreoretinal surgery or years after intracapsular cataract extraction. Second, the patient is pseudophakic with dislocated intraocular lens or even dislocated capsular bag-intraocular lens-complex., as seen in Figs. 1 and 2, sometimes with capsular tension ring in place. Even more complicated if previous secondary implantation with intraocular (transiridal or transscleral) suturing was performed. Last the vitreoretinal surgeon could recognize the dislocation during intraocular surgery (preexisting or caused by the surgeon himself) complicating the surgery and may require intraoperative repair.

Fixation of intraocular lenses in case of insufficient or no capsular support is challenging and requires a large augmentarium of techniques to solve different situations [1–22].

Supplementary Information The online version contains supplementary material available at https://doi.org/10.1007/978-3-031-32855-8_2.

G. B. Scharioth (✉)
Aurelios Augenzentrum, Erlbruch 34-36, 45657 Recklinghausen, Germany
e-mail: Gabor.scharioth@augenzentrum.org

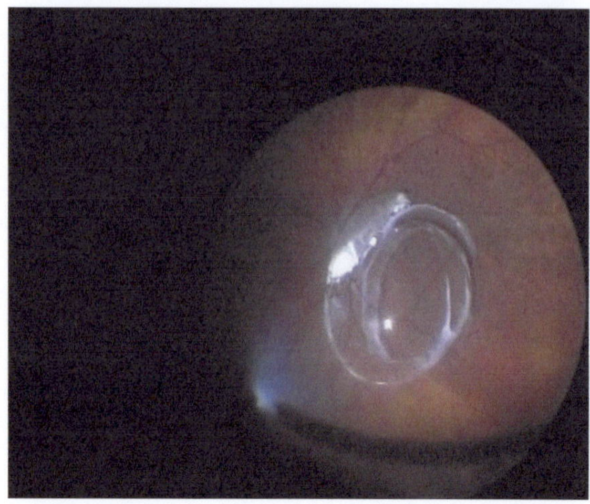

Fig. 1 Intraoperative appearance of completely luxated capsular bag—intraocular lens—capsular tension ring—complex ten years after uneventful phacoemulsification and in-the-bag PCIOL implantation in an eye with pseudoexfoliation syndrome

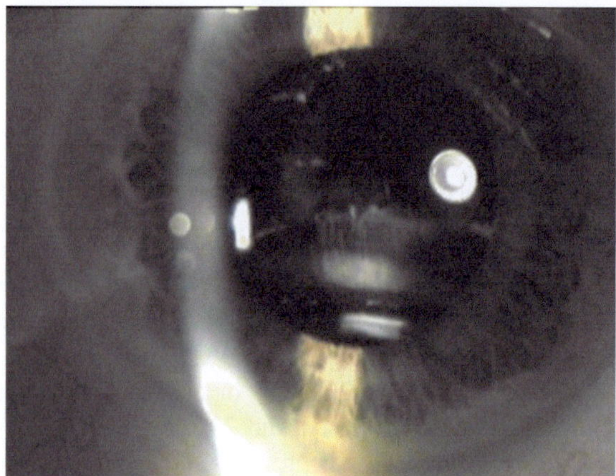

Fig. 2 Inferior dislocated capsular bag—intraocular lens—complex (Sunset syndrome) 8 years after uneventful phacoemulsification and in-the-bag PCIOL implantation in an eye with pseudoexfoliation syndrome

Since the introduction of intraocular lenses in cataract surgery by Sir Harold Ridley this became standard of care in late 80s. Whenever possible in-the-bag implantation with overlapping continuous curvilinear capsulorrhexis is preferable. But various IOL models and fixation sites and techniques are recommended for difficult situations.

Anterior chamber lenses were used for many years because of relatively easy implantation technique even in the total absence of capsular support. But the fixation in the anterior chamber angle may cause glaucoma and chronic irritation to iris. Furthermore long term endothelial cell loss with corneal decompensation is reported for angle fixated intraocular lenses as well as for iris claw lenses fixed to anterior surface, a technique introduced by Jan Worst almost thirty years ago. Both require relatively large incisions up to 6.5 mm. For iris claw lenses Uveitis-Glaucoma-Hemmorrhage Syndrome is reported and late dislocations may occur.

Anyway if someone would use this type of lens we recommend the retropupillary reverse implantation technique [21]. This is much more convenient because it prevents contact to corneal endothelium intraoperatively i.e. during fluid-air-exchange during a pars plana vitrectomy and postoperatively due to eye rubbing, blinking etc. Iris fixated IOL tend to cause IOL wobbeling with optical side effects and unstable vision. Some Surgeons prefer iris-sutured intraocular lenses. This could cause pupil ovalisation and iris chaffing with uveitis and/or pigment dispersion and secondary complications like chronic inflammation and secondary glaucoma. Anyway these techniques need sufficient iris stroma for fixation and cannot be used in aniridic patients.

We are convinced that the best place for fixation of intraocular lens in the absence of sufficient zonular/capsular support is the sclera. It is the strongest intraocular tissue, mainly avascular and does not tend to inflammation. Vitreoretinal surgeons know for decades that implants and explants for retinal procedures are well tolerated over a long period of time. In moderately damaged zonular apparatus we are using for many years capsular bag refixation techniques with modified capsular tension rings (s.c. Cionni ring) or Ahmed segments (both Morcher, Germany). These implants are positioned in the capsular bag and have an extra eyelet which is positioned on the anterior surface of the anterior capsule and fixed with a 10×0 or 9×0 Prolene suture transsclerally into the ciliary sulcus. This technique is difficult and needs an intact capsulorrhexis. Furthermore capsular bag cleaning is diminished. This tends to cause early secondary cataract and capsular fibrosis with rhexis phimosis. For more severe luxated capsular bags or for fixation of intraocular lenses in the absence of sufficient support the haptic of the intraocular lens could be knotted to a 10×0 or 9×0 Prolene suture and fixed to the scleral wall. Many variations of transscleral suture fixation are reported and this techniques are used worldwide because small incision techniques can be used, intraocular lens is positioned more physiologically in the posterior chamber and standard lenses could be used. In case of dislocated intraocular lens this could be refixated by intraoperative haptic externalization for knot fixation to the haptic and transsclerally suturefixation without need for intraocular lens explantation. A fibrosed capsular bag esp. if with capsular tension ring in place can easily refixated with double armed 10×0 or 9×0 Prolene suture to the ciliary sulcus. The first needle is passed through the capsule catching the haptic and/or capsular tension ring and passed through the sclera while the second needle is just placed above the bag through the sclera. The so created suture loop will hold the bag after knotting to the sclera. Usually more than one sclerafixation is necessary to stabilize the whole bag. Recently Richard Hoffmann reported a technique for transcleral suturefixation without opening of conjunctiva [22]. Here the pockets for suture knots are prepared from the limbus intrascleral towards the sclera, a double armed suture is used and stitched 1.5 mm postlimbal through the scleral pockets and conjunctiva, needles are cut off and the sutures are catched with a hook from the limbus. Then the suture is knotted and the ends are buried into the scleral pocket.

However centration of suturefixated intraocular lenses is difficult and lens tilt is a common problem. This will result in internal astigmatism and inconvenient refractive outcome. Fixation into the ciliary sulcus without capsular and zonular support is difficult and malpositioning may result in chronic irritation to ciliary body and/or iris with secondary complications. Good long term stability is reported but late dislocations due to suture biodegradation may occur and require reinterventions [23–27] There is a long learning curve for suturefixation techniques and outcome is very much depending on surgeons experience. Furthermore there could be a need for special intraocular lens, which may not be available everywhere and prompt, need extra costs and logistics, adapted biometry etc.

For these reasons we were searching for technique for intraocular lens fixation in the absence of sufficient capsular support which uses a standard foldable intraocular lens, sclerafixation, is independent from iris changes and the amount of zonular/capsular damage, sutureless, reduces the contact to uveal tissue and could be standardized.

In 2006 we performed the first intrascleral haptic fixation of a standard three piece intraocular lens and reported the surgical technique in 2007 [28].

This sutureless technique for fixation of a posterior chamber intraocular lens is using permanent incarceration of the haptics in a scleral tunnel parallel to the limbus. After peritomy the eye is stabilized either by pars plana infusion (i.e. 25G) or by anterior chamber maintainer. We try to prevent any diathermy of episcleral vessels to reduce the risk for scleral atrophy. Two straight sclerotomies ab externo are prepared with a sharp 23G cannula or 23G MVR blade about 1.5 mm postlimbal exactly 180° from each other and directed towards the centre of the globe, as seen in Figs. 3, 4 and 5. Then new cannulas are used to create a limbus-parallel tunnel at about 50% of scleral thickness, starting from inside the ciliary sulcus sclerotomies, as seen in Fig. 6, and ending with externalisation of the cannula after 2.0–3.0 mm, as seen in Fig. 7. A standard 3-piece IOL with a haptic design

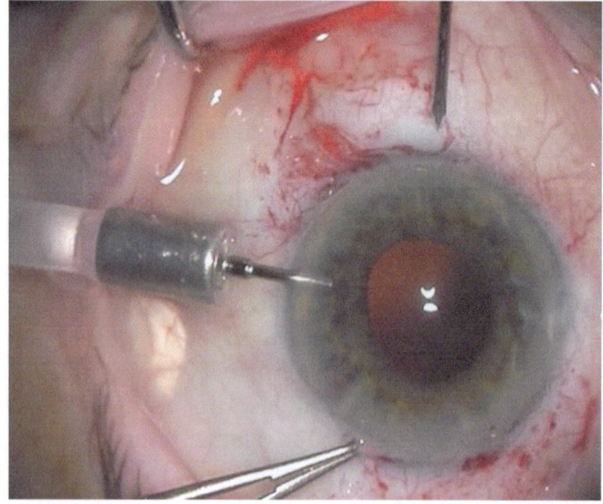

Fig. 3 After peritotomy, anterior chamber maintainer (25G infusion line) placed in a micro side port, 23G or 24G sharp cannula is used to create a straight ciliary sulcus sclerotomy 1.5 to 2.0 mm postlimbal

Fig. 4 Second sclerotomy shall be placed exactly 180°, alternatively a corneal marker could be used

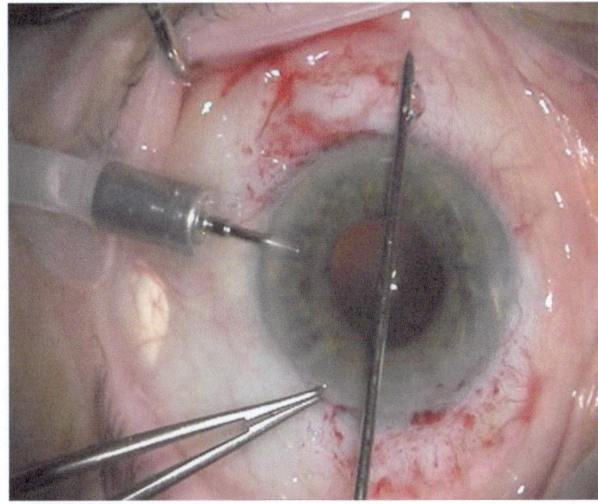

Fig. 5 A 23G or 24G sharp cannula is used to create a straight ciliary sulcus sclerotomy 1.5 to 2.0 mm postlimbal exactly opposite to the first

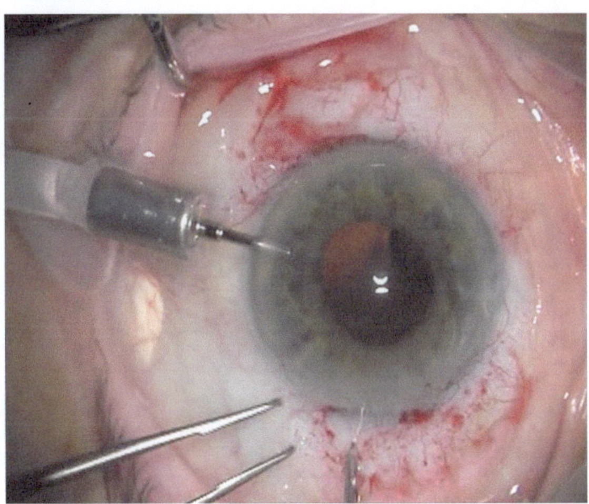

fitting to the diameter of ciliary sulcus is implanted with an injector, and the tailing haptic is fixated in the corneal incision, as seen in Figs. 8 and 9. The leading haptic is then grasped at its tip with a special straight 25G forceps (Scharioth IOL fixation forceps 1286.SFD, DORC Int., The Netherlands), pulled through the sclerotomy and left externalized, as seen in Figs. 10, 11, 12 and 13.

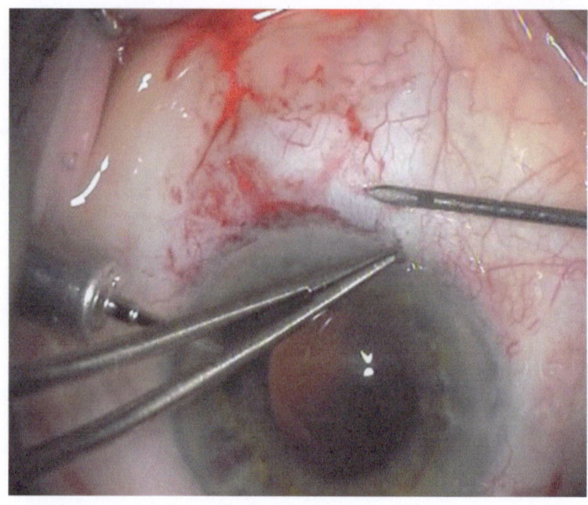

Fig. 6 Intrascleral limbusparallel tunnel is created counterclockwise with a 23G or 24G sharp cannula

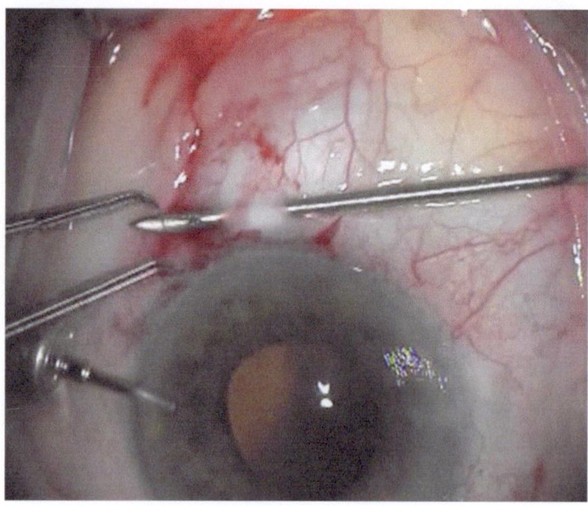

Fig. 7 After 2–3 mm the cannula is externalized and withdrawn, same is performed on opposite sclerotomy side

Fig. 8 Injector assisted implantation of foldable IOL

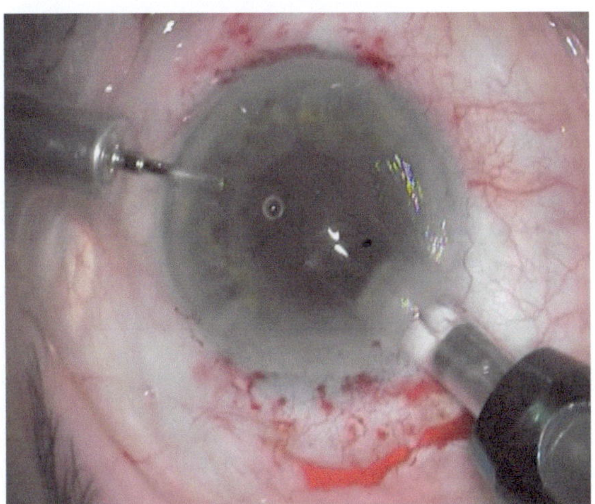

Fig. 9 IOL implanted with leading haptic behind iris and trailing haptic fixed inside the corneal incision, continious irrigation is mandatory to prevent collapse of the eye with haptic sleapage from the main incision

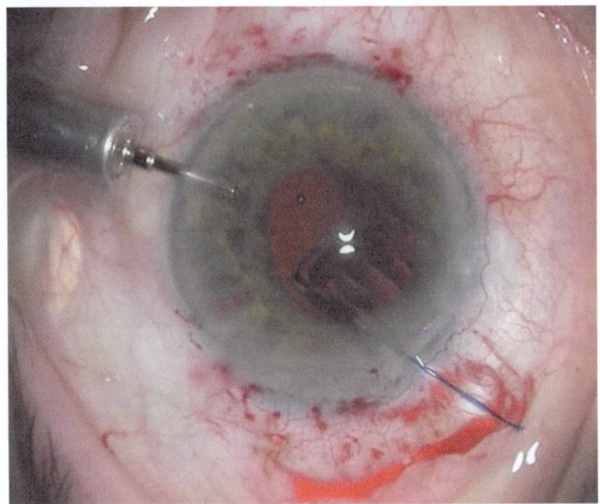

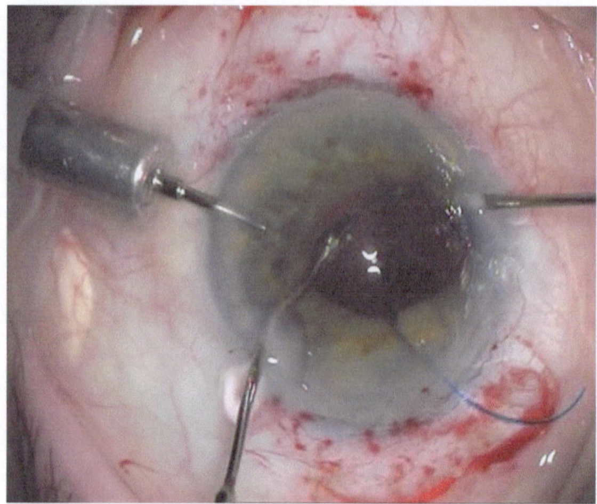

Fig. 10 "Hand shake maneuver" using Scharioth forceps, IOL haptic is grasped with right hand first and presented to grasp the haptic with left hand, then right hand forceps is removed from anterior chamber and introduced through opposite ciliary sulcus sclorotomy

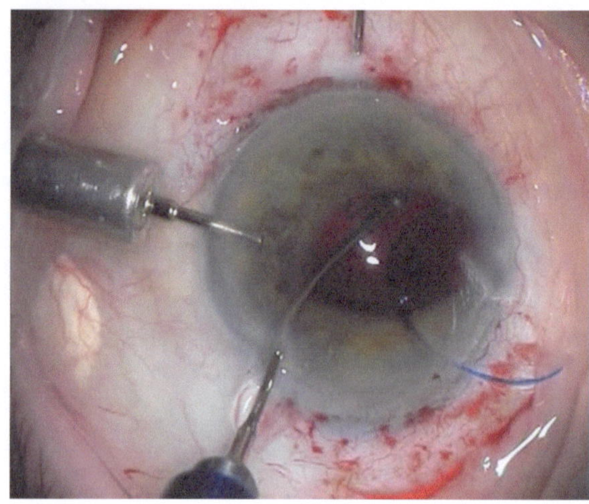

Fig. 11 "Hand shake maneuver" using Scharioth forceps, IOL is still hold with left hand forceps, second forceps is grasping the very tip of IOL haptic, then left hand releases haptic and while right hand forceps is withdrawn the haptic is externalized through ciliary sulcus sclerotomy

Fig. 12 Leading haptic externalized through ciliary sulcus sclerotomy, trailing haptic still in fixated corneal incision

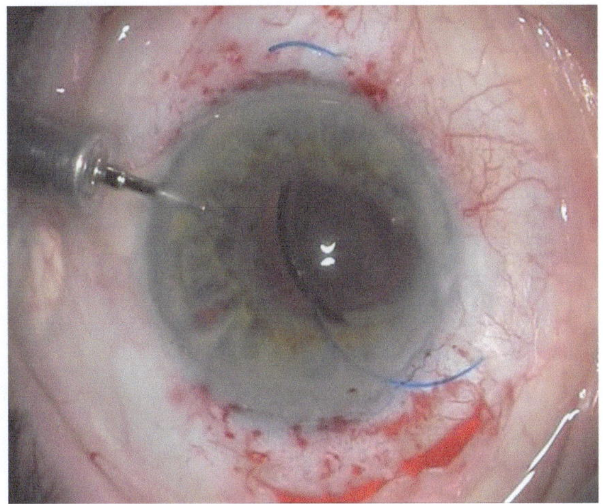

Fig. 13 Both haptics externalized after same "hand shake maneuver" is performed with trailing haptic

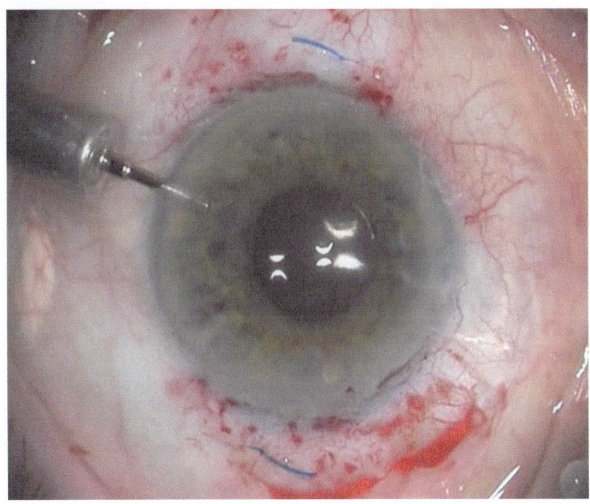

With the curved Scharioth forceps then the haptic is grasped at its tip, introduced into the intrascleral tunnel and pushed through, as seen in Fig. 14. Then the haptic is released, as seen in Fig. 15, forceps is turned, closed and pulled back leaving the haptic in the sclera (pushing technique). Turning the forceps after release of haptic will reduce the risk of pulling the haptic while retracting the forceps from the intrascleral tunnel. Alternatively one can introduce the Scharioth forceps from the distal end of the intrascleral tunnel until it becomes visible in the sclerotomy, then the haptic tip is grasped and pulled in the scleral tunnel (pulling technique). The same maneuvers are performed with the tailing haptic. The ends of the haptic are left in the tunnel, as seen in Fig. 16, to prevent foreign body sensation, erosion of the conjunctiva and to reduce the risk for inflammation. The sclerotomies are checked for leakage and if necessary sutured.

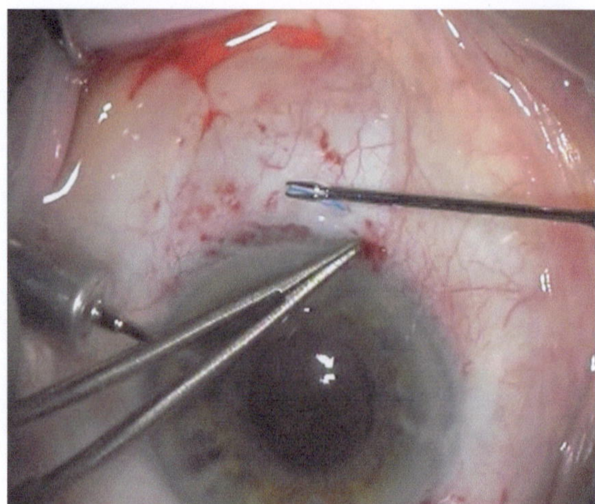

Fig. 14 Curved Scharioth forceps is used to grasp the very tip of one haptic, then the haptic is pushed a bit backwards until it can be introduced into the limbusparallel intrascleral tunnel

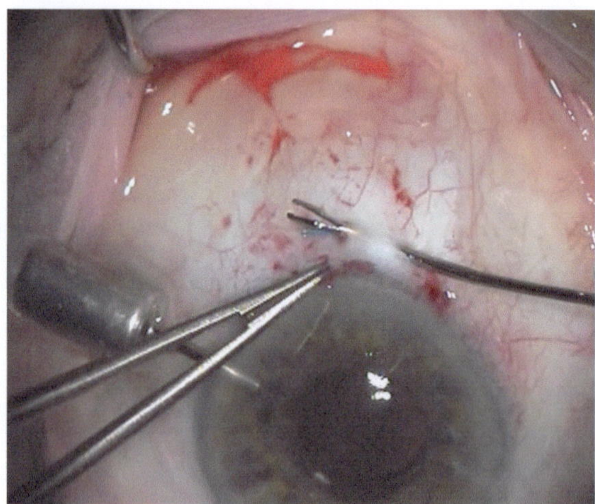

Fig. 15 Forceps holding the haptic is pushed through the limbusparallel intrascleral tunnel, after tip is externalized the haptic is released, forceps is then turn and closed before withdrawn, this will reduce risk of catching the haptic

Some surgeons use other forceps for this technique (e.g. Grieshaber® serrated forceps 25G, Alcon, USA). This will work but as the forceps is straight intrascleral haptic implantation can become quite difficult in deep seated eyes, small lid opening and/or patients with big nose. We therefore developed a set of two forseps. One is longer and straight to externalize the haptic through sulcus cilliary sclerotomies and also to be able to grasp dislocated IOL even in high myopic eyes. The other forceps is shorter and better for manipulations in the anterior segment / chamber during hand shake and for the haptic insertion into the limbus parallel intrascleral tunnel (Scharioth IOL fixation forceps 1286.SFD, DORC Int., The Netherlands).

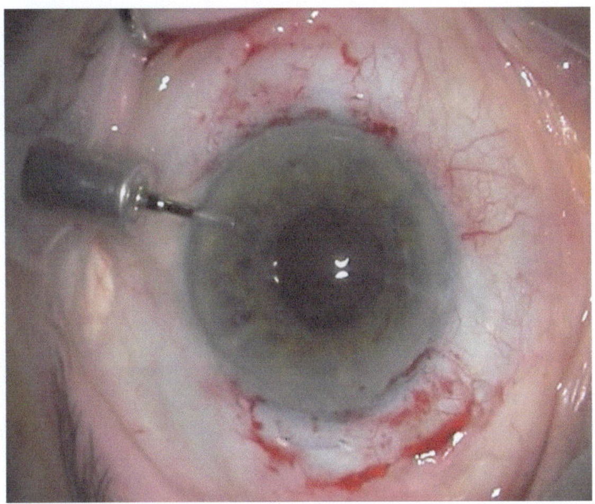

Fig. 16 Both haptics are placed intrasclerally, it is important that the haptic is completely covered by sclera

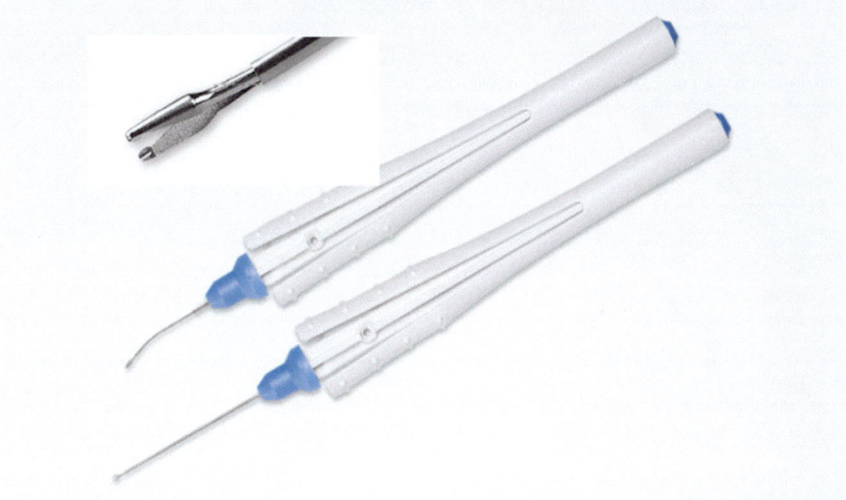

Following this described technique and three piece IOL could be implanted and stably fixated in eyes without sufficient capsular support. Figure 17 shows slit lamp photo 8 years postoperative with no signs of erosion or inflammation. The haptic is well positioned and could be seen shining through sclera and conjunctiva. Postoperative OCT could be used to proof intrascleral positioning of the haptics, as seen in Fig. 18.

We have used this technique in hundreds of eyes over the past twelve years. Our standard IOL were Sensar AR40e (AMO, USA) and Acrysof (Alcon, USA) but any three piece IOL sufficient for sulcus fixation should work. In 2010 we reported our interim results of a European multicenter study. We had 4 haptic dislocations

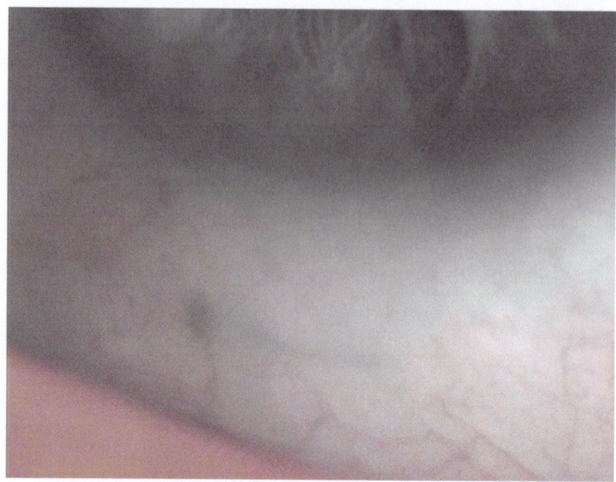

Fig. 17 Slit lamp photo 8 years postoperative after sutureless intrascleral haptic fixation, no sign of inflammation or scleral erosion in the area of incarcerated haptic

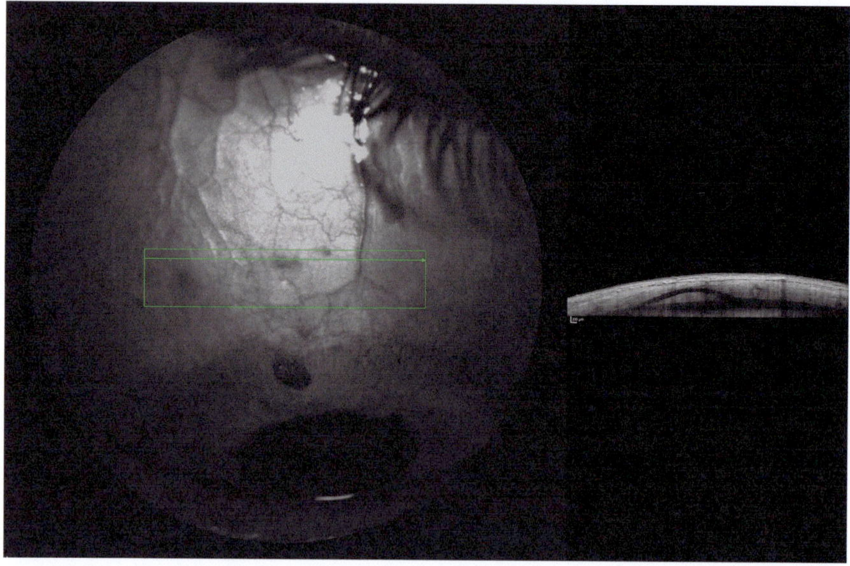

Fig. 18 Postoperative anterior segment OCT, left image showing intrascleral placement of IOL haptic without scleral changes or signs of leakage

which could be reimplanted and one transient vitreous hemorrhage. These complications occurred all in the first ten cases and in first 4 postoperative weeks [29]. Some young patients with floppy iris showed postoperative recurrent iris capture which disappeared after NdYAG laser iridotomy or better surgical iridectomy. If this condition is anticipated we suggest intraoperative iridectomy with the vitreous cutter. Also some patients show reverse pupillary block with iris sticking to the IOL surface and very deep anterior chamber. In this case an iridectomy with the

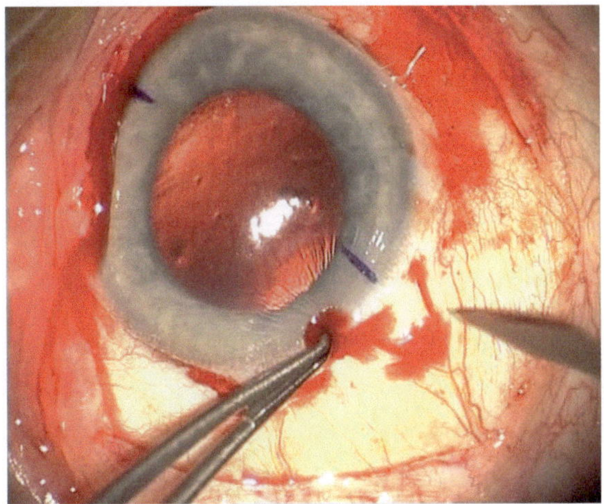

Fig. 19 Glued IOL technique, preparation of scleral flap, note corneal marks to improve location

vitreous cutter is solving the problem. In our experience anterior chamber depth will immediately return to normal and a repeated inflation of the AC should not cause a recurrent reverse pupillary block.

For PCIOL calculation we use the SRK-T formula and the same A-constant as for in-the-bag implantation.

Later a variation of our technique was introduced by Agarwal [30]. After peritotomy two half thickness scleral flaps are created postlimbal exactly 180° to each other, as seen in Fig. 19. Then straight sclerotomies are prepared, Fig. 20, and the IOL haptics are externalized, as seen in Fig. 22. Originally Agarwal left the haptics under the scleral flap and closed with fibrin glue. Over the last years he recommends to create a intrascleral tunnel counterclockwise at the edge of the scleral bed, as seen in Fig. 21. This tunnel (so called Scharioth tuck) is prepared with a 27G needle and the haptik is then introduced with the help of a tying forceps, as seen in Fig. 23. Then scleral flap and conjunctiva are closed with fibrin glue (Fig. 24).

Totan and Karadag introduced another modification of intrascleral haptic fixation [31]. With the help of a 23G or 25G transconjunctival trocar system a short intrascleral tunnel is created. Then the tip of the haptic is grasped and while externalized the trocar cannula is removed. The haptic is left in a short intrascleral tunnel. The reduced surgical time and trauma seems to be advantageous but has to weighted with an increased risk for postoperative IOL dislocation. Furthermore as the intrascleral haptic fixation is very short an intraoperative fine tuning (final minimal repositioning of the IOL) is not possible. The authors report in a small study with 29 eyes that there was no significant difference between this technique and the original Scharioth technique [32].

Later Yamane et al. recommended the so called double needle technique. Here a longer transconjunctival tunnel is created with sharp 30G needle. After temporary externalisation of the haptics these are cauterized at its tip to form a small bulb.

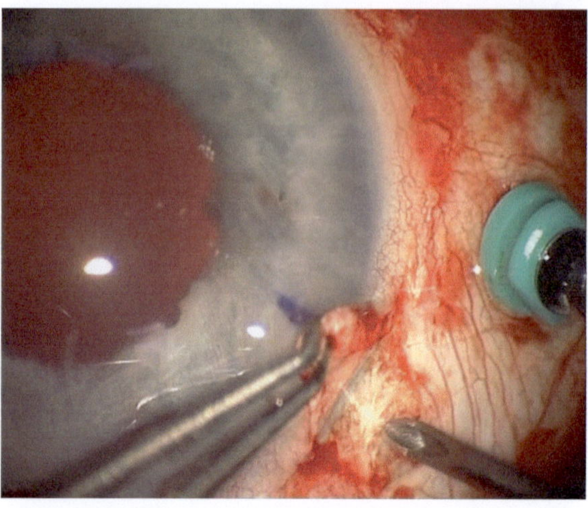

Fig. 20 Glued IOL technique, under flap ciliary sulcus sclerotomy with 23G sharp cannula

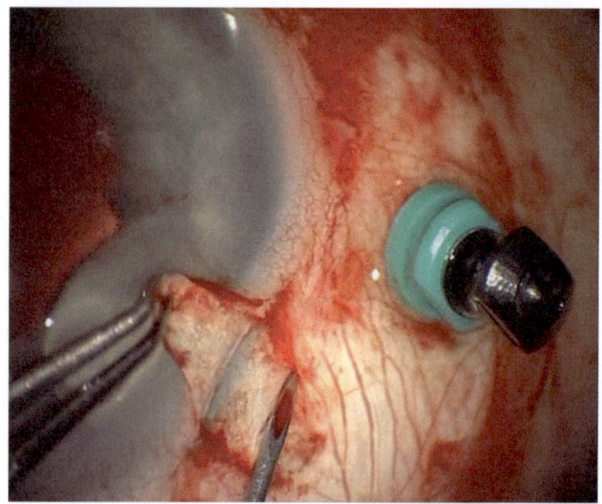

Fig. 21 Glued IOL technique, Scharioth tuck is performed with 27G sharp cannula at the margin of scleral bed

Then the haptics are positioned intrascleral. This should reduce the risk for haptic dislocation [33].

Over the past decade we have operated on many eyes with dislocated capsular bag-IOL-complex with single piece IOL. Initially we removed the whole complex and followed by implantation of a new three piece IOL as described. Later we started to refixate the single piece IOL if it was a Acrysof® (Alcon, USA). Herefore pars plana vitrectomy and a complete capsulectomy was performed. If a capsular tension ring was in place this has to be explanted through a side port incision. Ciliary sulcus peritotomy was performed with a 23G cannula as described. But then a 20G cannula was used to create a short intrascleral tunnel. We implanted only the thick knob (very distal end) of the Acrysof® haptic, as seen in Fig. 25, into the intrascleral pocket. Here it is very important not to twist the haptic as

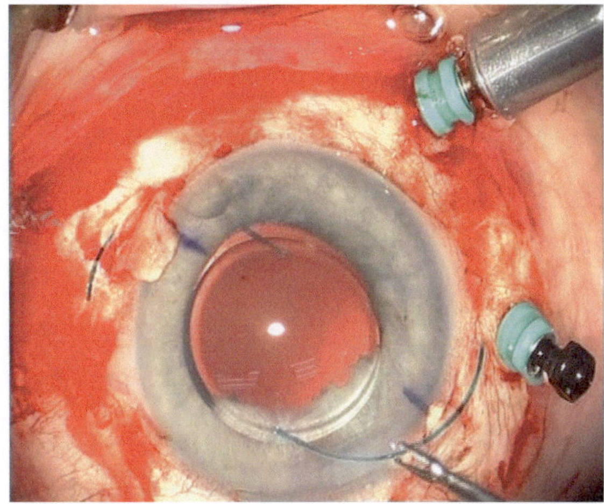

Fig. 22 Glued IOL technique, leading haptic externalized, trailing haptic prior to implantation

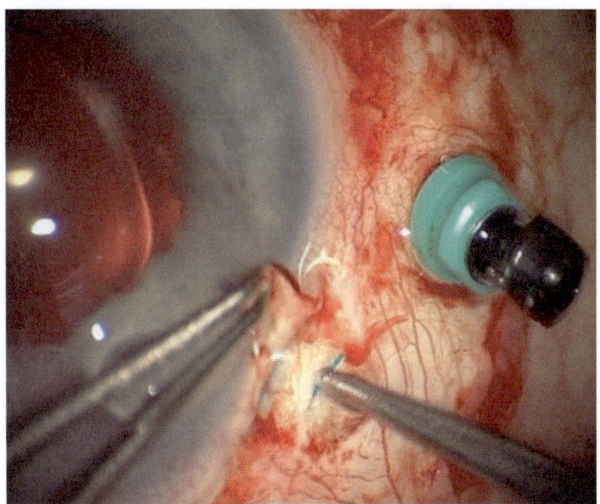

Fig. 23 Glued IOL technique, haptic is grasped with a tying forceps and implanted into the Scharioth tuck

this would easily induce an IOL tilt with lens induced astigmatism. After this initial positive experience we use this single piece IOL also if a refractive power over +30 D is needed. Postoperative controls and OCT imaging showed complete intrascleral positioning of the square edged haptic, as seen in Figs. 26 and 27.

With a longer follow up we saw that about 50% of cases a transscleral and transconjunctival haptic erosion developed, as seen in Fig. 28. In these cases we reopened the conjunctiva and trimmed the haptic with scissors. Then sclera was mobilized, sutured over the haptic to recover and conjunctiva refixated, as seen in Fig. 29. In no case an explantation was needed or a recurrent erosion occurred. Later we modified the technique and trimmed immediately the haptic. With this thinned haptic no erosion or other complication was observed on long term. Still

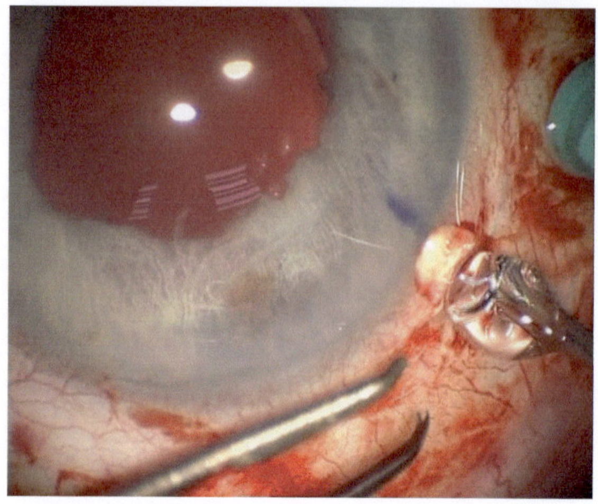

Fig. 24 Glued IOL technique, fibrin glue is applied under the scleral flap and then later to close the conjunctiva

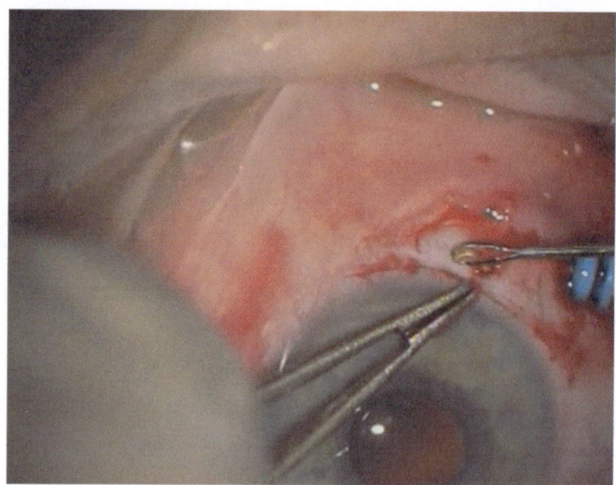

Fig. 25 Haptic of a single piece Acrysof® just prior to intrascleral implantation

we use Acrysof single piece IOL only for cases that require implantation of IOL with more than +30 dioptres or multifocal IOL.

In young patients subluxated or even luxated crystalline lens after severe trauma, as seen in Fig. 30, or Marfan syndrome implantation of a multifocal IOL might be indicated. We reported in 2011 on our positive initial results [34]. Three piece PCIOL (ReZoom® and Tecnis® Multifocal, AMO, Santa Ana, USA) have been used with described technique for sutureless intrascleral haptic fixation. Figure 31 showes such a multifocal PCIOL before and Fig. 32 after pupilloplasty for traumatic mydriasis. To improve refractive outcome in case of postoperative ammetropia laserrefractive surgery (BIOPTICS) could be used. We recommend LASEK or PRK because the use of a suction ring during LASIK could weaken

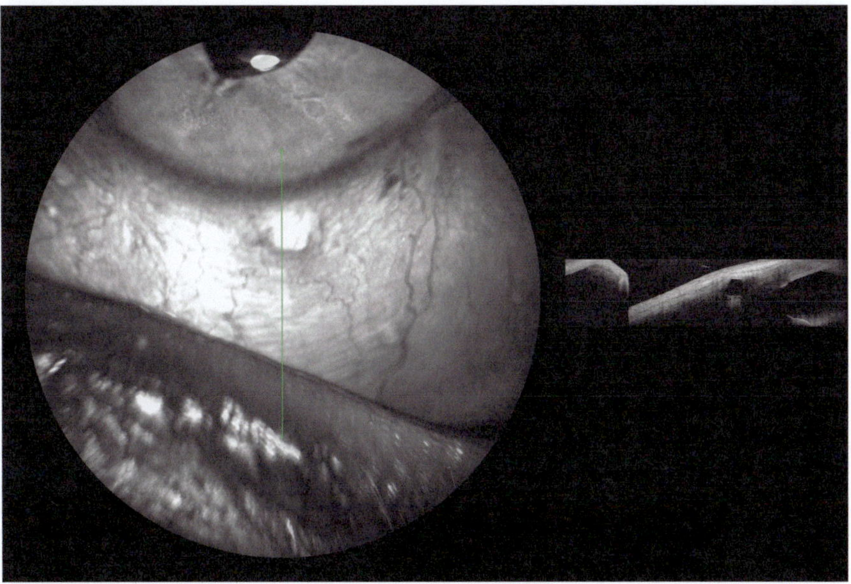

Fig. 26 Postoperative anterior segment OCT, left image showing intrascleral placement of IOL haptic without scleral changes or signs of leakage, note square edge haptic

Fig. 27 Intrascleral fixated haptic of an Acrysof® single piece IOL 24 months postoperative

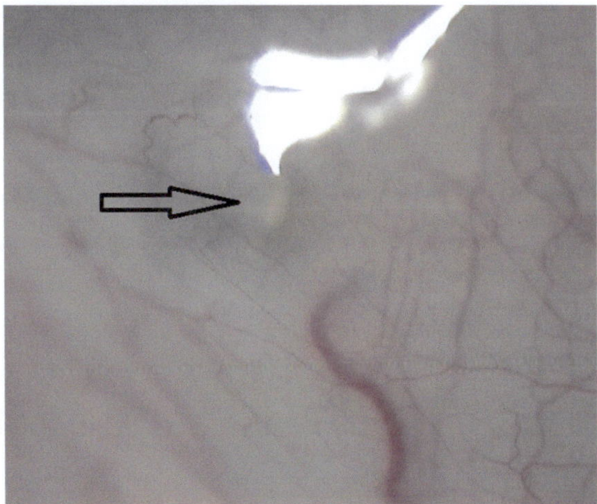

the intrascleral fixation. In some patients a corneal wavefront guided laserrefractive surgery could be used to reduce higher order aberrations. Even many years later these IOL stay stable and well centered, as seen in Fig. 33.

Currently most three piece IOL with multifocal optics are not available anymore. So that we recently have started to implant single piece hydrophobic

Fig. 28 Transsscleral and
transconjunctival erosion of
square edged haptic
14 months postoperative

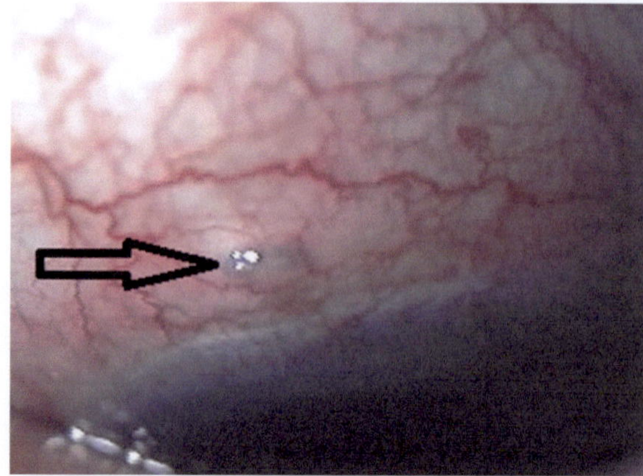

Fig. 29 Same eye after
revision with haptic
trimming, scleral suture to
cover haptic end and
conjunctival revision

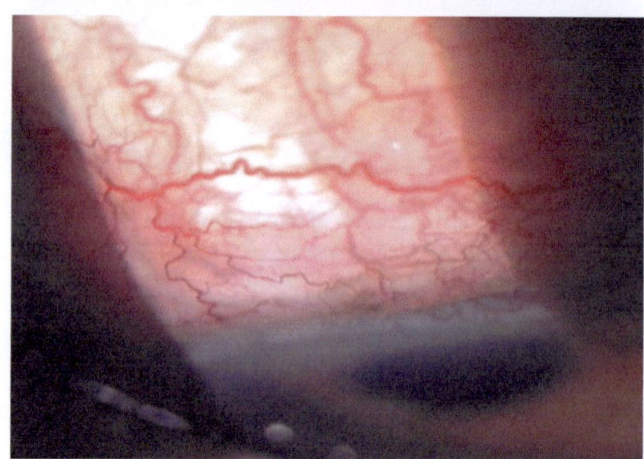

Fig. 30 Preoperative
situation in a case after severe
blunt trauma, 4 weeks after
trauma hypermature cataract,
severe subluxation of
crystalline lens and vitreous
prolapse in anterior chamber

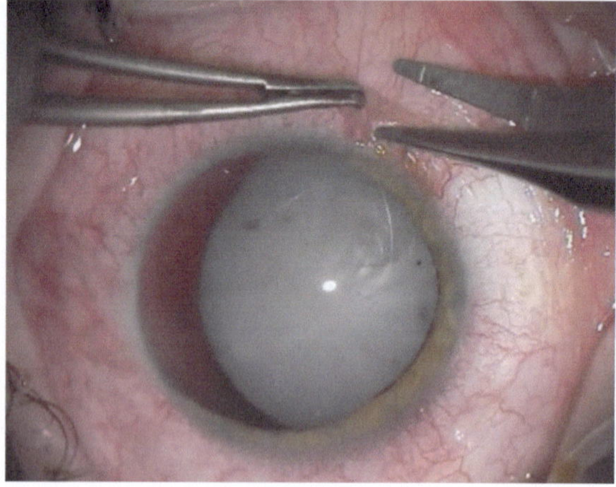

Fig. 31 Intrascleral haptic fixation of multifocal PCIOL (ReZoom® Multifocal, AMO, Santa Ana, USA) 6 weeks postoperative prior to iris reconstruction in a 34 years old male after lensectomy and pars plana vitrectomy for traumatic subluxation of a hypermature cataract and retinal detachment after severe blunt trauma, note extreme posttraumatic mydriasis

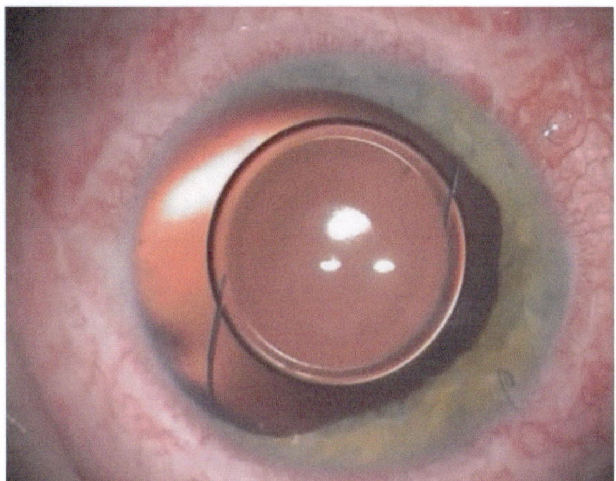

Fig. 32 Patient after iridoplastic with iris stretching and multiple iris sutures, final best uncorrected visual acuity for distance and near 0.8

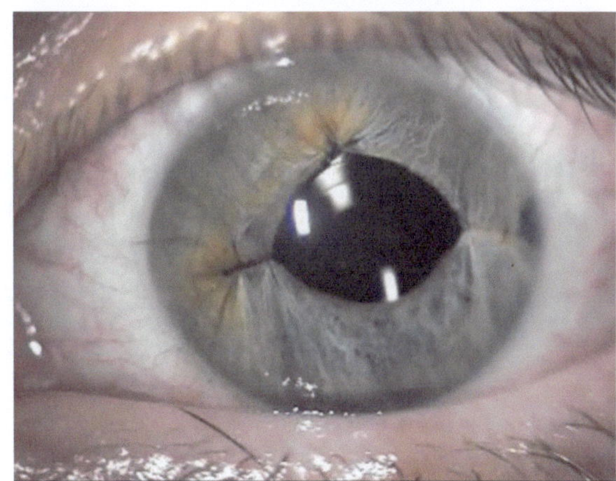

Fig. 33 Intrascleral haptic fixated multifocal PCIOL (ReZoom® Multifocal, AMO, Santa Ana, USA) in a young patient with Marfan Syndrome after postoperative corneal wavefront guided LASEK for improved refractive result, final best uncorrected visual acuity for distance and near 0.8

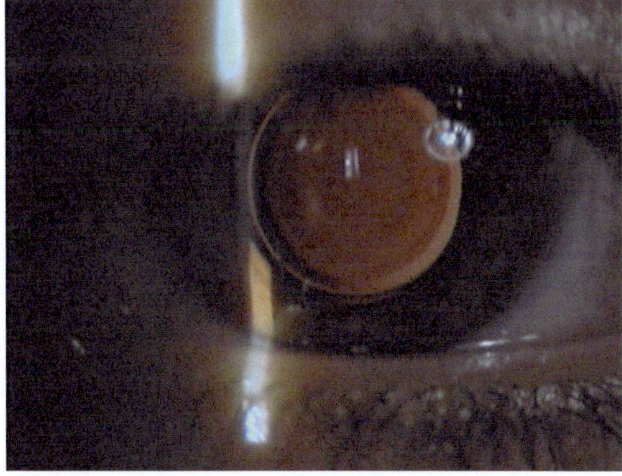

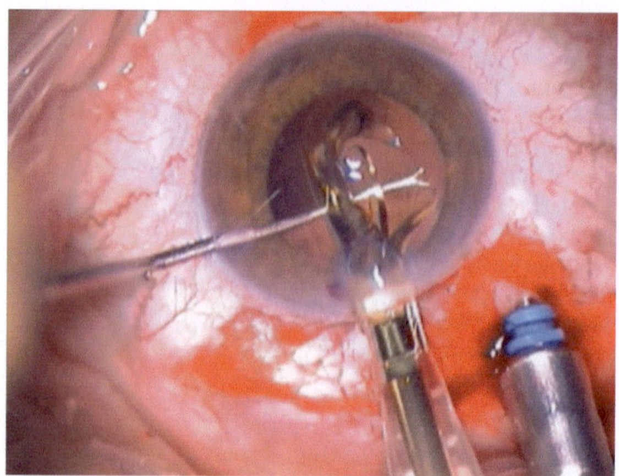

Fig. 34 Injector assisted implantation of single piece Acrysof® Panoptix into anterior chamber, note second instrument that is placed under the IOL to prevent dislocation into vitreous cavity, pars plana infusion placed to ensure stable intraocular pressure and to prevent collapse of the eye

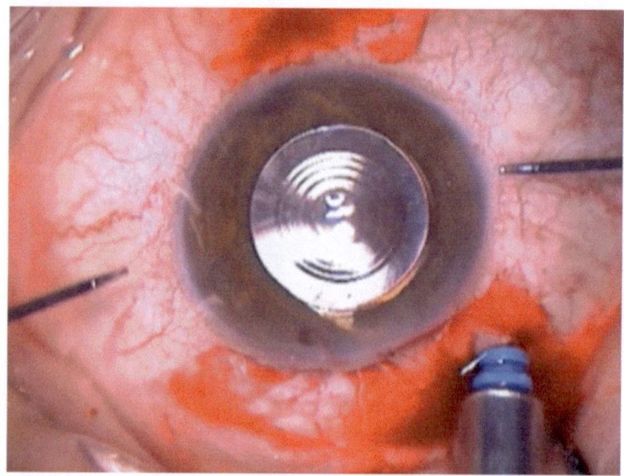

Fig. 35 Stable situation with single piece IOL placed in anterior chamber, two forceps (Scharioth forceps) used for hand shake technique

acrylic lenses (AcrySof® IQ PanOptix®, Alcon, USA) using a 20G intrascleral limbusparallel tunnel, as seen in Figs. 34, 35, 36, 37, 38 and 39.

In case of Aniridia we combined also IOL implantation with intrascleral haptic fixation and additional implantation of suture fixated artificial iris Human Optics, Germany). This is a challenging surgery. We prefer to first implant the IOL and then implant and suture the artificial iris, as seen in Figs. 40, 41 and 42. By this the main incision could be kept around 3.0 mm. Another option would be to suture the artificial iris to the IOL haptics and fold the whole complex with a forceps for implantation. Here a much bigger incision is needed.

Management of secondary implantation or refixation of dislocated intraocular lenses with the use of scleral tunnel fixation of the haptic is less technically demanding because it stabilizes the intraocular lens in the posterior chamber without difficult suturing procedures and uses a real microsurgical approach if injector assisted IOL implantation is used in combination with 25G or even 27G vitrectomy system. Incarcerating a longer part of the haptic stabilizes the axial position

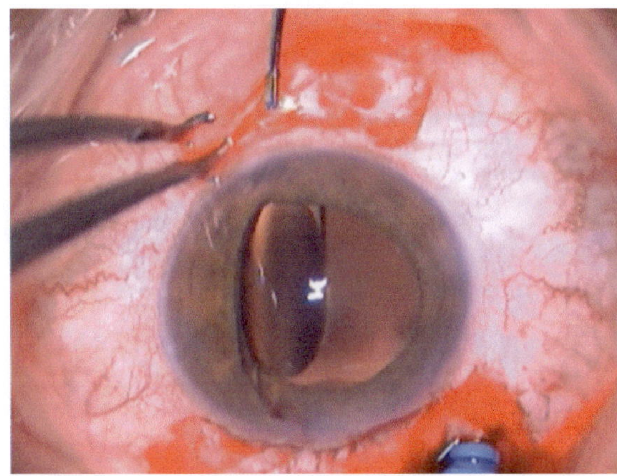

Fig. 36 One haptic externalized through ciliary sulcus sclerotomy and grasped with Scharioth forceps, note twisted IOL

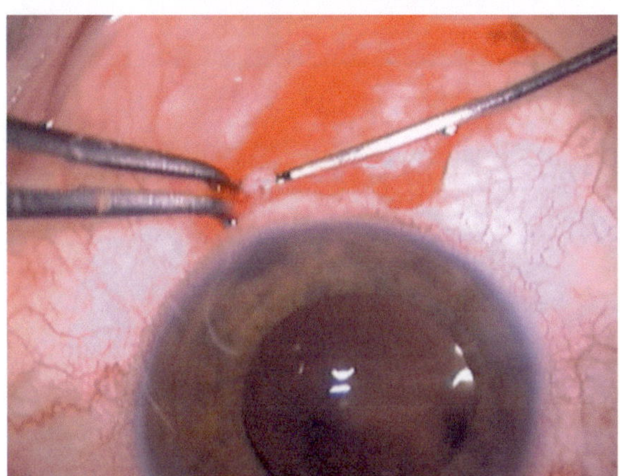

Fig. 37 Implantation of Acrysof® IOL haptic into intrascleral pocket/tunnel, IOL position immediately improved

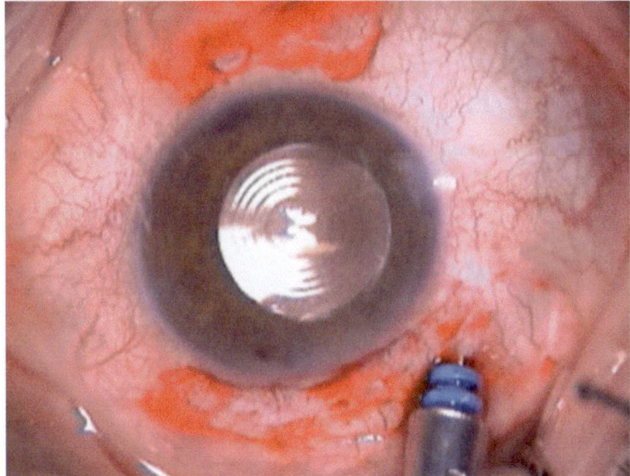

Fig. 38 Final intraoperative situs with single piece Acrysof® Panoptix IOL in place, note excellent centration without tilt

Fig. 39 Postoperative photo in retroillumination with well centered MFIOL with intrascleral haptic fixation (Acrysof® Panoptix IOL) one year after surgery

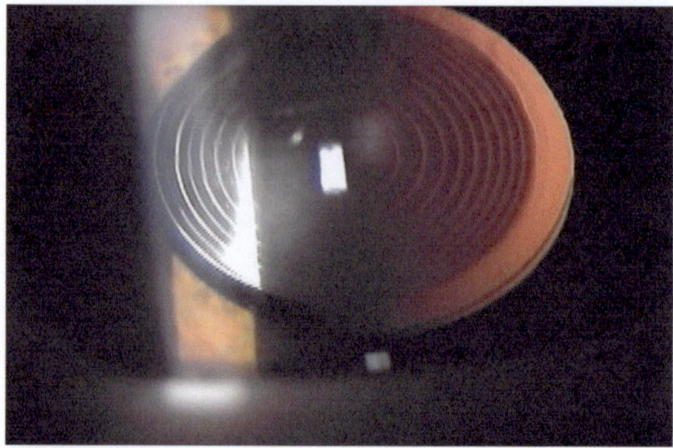

Fig. 40 Aniridic and aphakic eye 30 years after severe trauma

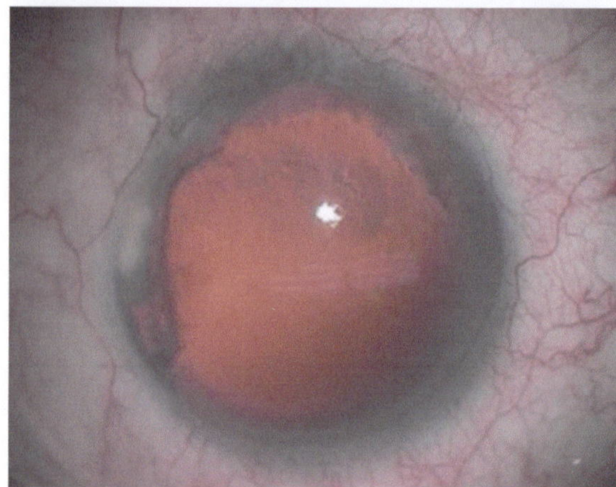

Fig. 41 Intraoperative situation after implantation of a three piece IOL with intrascleral haptic fixation

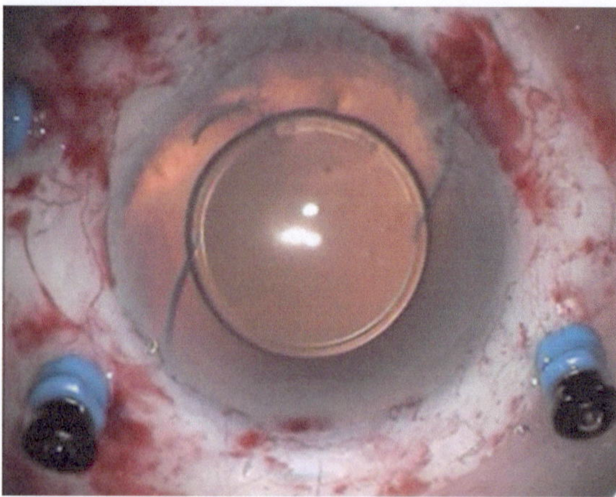

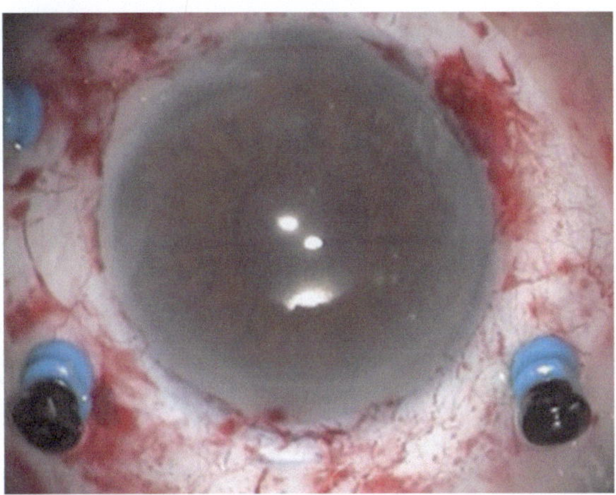

Fig. 42 Same eye after implantation and suture fixation of artificial iris

of the PC IOL, which should decrease the incidence of IOL tilt. More than fifteen years follow up with only minimal complication after the early postoperative period and learning period for this procedure seems to indicate the excellent long term stability of intraocular lenses fixated with this technique. In our opinion the only possible contraindications are chronic scleritis or scleromalacia, but these are very rare conditions.

However cataract and vitreoretinal surgeons should be familiar with different techniques for fixation of intraocular lenses because we will be faced with situation were an intraocular lens is already implanted and requires secondary intervention. In future urgent phacoemulsification problems like dropped nucleus less often will need revision, but more often we will see eyes with late dislocation of the entire capsular bag after primary uneventful cataract surgery because of chronic ongoing disease like pseudoexfoliation syndrome. We should be able to select a less demanding and traumatizing technique which gives a great chance that no further intervention is necessary.

References

1. Anand R, Bowman RW. Simplified technique for suturing dislocated posterior chamber intraocular lens to the ciliary sulcus [letter]. Arch Ophthalmol. 1990;108:1205–6.
2. Azar DT, Wiley WF. Double-knot transscleral suture fixation technique for displaced intraocular lenses. Am J Ophthalmol. 1999;128:644–6.
3. Bloom SM, Wyszynski RE, Brucker AJ. Scleral fixation suture for dislocated posterior chamber intraocular lens. Ophthalmic Surg. 1990;21:851–4.
4. Chan CK. An improved technique for management of dislocated posterior chamber implants. Ophthalmology. 1992;99:51–7.
5. Chang S. Perfluorocarbon liquids in vitreoretinal surgery. Int Ophthalmol Clin. 1992;32(2):153–63.

6. Chang S, Coll GE. Surgical techniques for repositioning a dislocated intraocular lens, repair of iridodialysis, and secondary intraocular lens implantation using innovative 25-gauge forceps. Am J Ophthalmol. 1995;119:165–74.

7. Fanous MM, Friedman SM. Ciliary sulcus fixation of a dislocated posterior chamber intraocular lens using liquid perfluorophenanthrene. Ophthalmic Surg. 1992;23:551–2.

8. Friedberg MA, Pilkerton AR. A new technique for repositioning and fixating a dislocated intraocular lens. Arch Ophthalmol. 1992;110:413–5.

9. Kokame GT, Yamamoto I, Mandel H. Scleral fixation of dislocated posterior chamber intraocular lenses; temporary haptic externalization through a clear corneal incision. J Cataract Refract Surg. 2004;30:1049–56.

10. Little BC, Rosen PH, Orr G, Aylward GW. Trans-scleral fixation of dislocated posterior chamber intraocular lenses using a 9/0 microsurgical polypropylene snare. Eye. 1993;7:740–3.

11. Maguire AM, Blumenkranz MS, Ward TG, Winkelman JZ. Scleral loop fixation for posteriorly dislocated intraocular lenses; operative technique and long-term results. Arch Ophthalmol. 1991;109:1754–8.

12. Nabors G, Varley MP, Charles S. Ciliary sulcus suturing of a posterior chamber intraocular lens. Ophthalmic Surg. 1990;21:263–5.

13. Schneiderman TE, Johnson MW, Smiddy WE, et al. Surgical management of posteriorly dislocated silicone plate haptic intraocular lenses. Am J Ophthalmol. 1997;123:629–35.

14. Shin DH, Hu BV, Hong YJ, Gibbs KA. Posterior chamber lens implantation in the absence of posterior capsular support [letter and reply by WJ Stark, GL Goodman, JD Gottsch]. Ophthalmic Surg. 1988;19:606–7.

15. Smiddy WE. Dislocated posterior chamber intraocular lens; a new technique of management. Arch Ophthalmol. 1989;107:1678–80.

16. Smiddy WE, Flynn HW Jr. Needle-assisted scleral fixation suture technique for relocating posteriorly dislocated IOLs [letter]. Arch Ophthalmol. 1993;111:161–2.

17. Smiddy WE, Ibanez GV, Alfonso E, Flynn HW Jr. Surgical management of dislocated intraocular lenses. J Cataract Refract Surg. 1995;21:64–9.

18. Thach AB, Dugel PU, Sipperley JO, et al. Outcome of sulcus fixation of dislocated posterior chamber intraocular lenses using temporary externalization of the haptics. Ophthalmology 2000;107:480–484 (discussion by WF Mieler, 485).

19. Koh HJ, Kim CY, Lim SJ, Kwon OW. Scleral fixation technique using 2 corneal tunnels for a dislocated intraocular lens. J Cataract Refract Surg. 2000;26:1439–41.

20. Lewis JS. Ab externo sulcus fixation. Ophthalmic Surg. 1991;22:692–5.

21. Mohr A, Hengerer F, Eckardt C. Retropupillare fixation der Irisklauenlinse bei Aphakie; Einjahresergebnisse einer neuen Implantationstechnik [Retropupillary fixation of the iris claw lens in aphakia; 1 year outcome of a new implantation technique.]. Ophthalmologe. 2002;99:580–3.

22. Hoffman RS, Fine I, Packar M. Scleral fixation without conjunctival dissection. J Cataract Refract Surg. 2006;32:1907–12.

23. Teichmann KD, Teichmann IAM. The torque and tilt gamble. J Cataract Refract Surg. 1997;23:413–8.

24. Por YM, Lavin MJ. Techniques of intraocular lens suspension in the absence of capsular/zonular support. Surv Ophthalmol. 2005;50:429–62.

25. Wagoner MD, Cox TA, Ariyasu RG, et al. Intraocular lens implantation in the absence of capsular support; a report by the American Academy of Ophthalmology. (Ophthalmic Technology Assessment) Ophthalmology 2003;110:840–859

26. Gross JG, Kokame GT, Weinberg DV. In-the-bag intraocular lens dislocation; the dislocated In-the-Bag Intraocular Len Study. Am J Ophthalmol. 2004;137:630–5.

27. Jehan FS, Mamalis N, Crandall AS. Spontaneous late dislocation of intraocular lens within the capsular bag in pseudoexfoliation patients. Ophthalmology. 2001;108:1727–31.

28. Gabor SG, Pavlidis MM. Sutureless intrascleral posterior chamber intraocular lens fixation. J Cataract Refract Surg. 2007;33:1851–4.

29. Scharioth GB, Prasad S, Georgalas I, Tatru C. Pavlidis M Intermediate results of sutureless intrascleral posterior chamber intraocular lens fixation. J Cataract Refract Surg. 2010;36:254–9.
30. Agarwal A, Kumar DA, Jacob S, Baid C, Agarwal A, Srinivasan. Fibrin glue-assisted sutureless posterior chamber intraocular lens implantation in eyes with deficient posterior capsules. J Cataract Refract Surg. 2008 Sep;34(9):1433–8
31. Totan Y, Karadag R. Trocar-assisted sutureless intrascleral posterior chamber foldable intraocular lens fixation. Eye (Lond). 2012;26(6):788–91.
32. Totan Y, Karadag R. Two techniques for sutureless intrascleral posterior chamber IOL fixation. J Refract Surg. 2013;29(2):90–4.
33. Yamane S, Inoue M, Arakawa A, Kadonosono K. Sutureless 27-gauge needle-guided intrascleral intraocular lens implantation with lamellar scleral dissection. Ophthalmology. 2014;121(1):61–6.
34. Pavlidis M, de Ortueta D, Scharioth GB. Bioptics in sutureless intrascleral multifocal posterior chamber intraocular lens fixation. J Refract Surg. 2011;27:386–8.

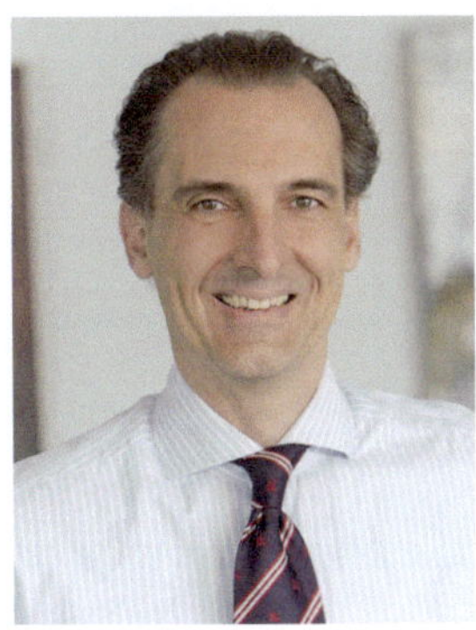

Gabor B. Scharioth graduated from Medical School in Humboldt University Berlin in 1993. During his residency program he was trained in Augentagesklinik Groß-Pankow, Campus Virchow of University Berlin and Aravind Eye Hospitals India. From 1998 He joined private practice in West Germany and founded Aurelios Eye Centers in 2002. Main focus in ophthalmic surgery are cataract surgery, vitreoretinal surgery, reconstructive/trauma surgery and modern glaucoma surgery. He has performed more than 40,000 surgeries during his career and trained many doctors around the world. He gave more than 300 scientific presentations at national and international conferences and performed more than 25 live surgeries at several international meetings around the world. Multiple scientific peer-reviewed publications are published and he was awarded several times at international meetings, incl. ASCRS, ESCRS, EVRS and DOC. He is member of several ophthalmic organisations, scientific and advisory boards. During his professional career he made several inventions like Scharioth Macula Lens for patients with advanced maculopathy, Glaucolight assisted canaloplasty, microscope mounted angle viewing system, Lightindentor for vitreoretinal surgery and intrascleral haptic fixation of PCIOL in absence of capsular support. He was principal investigator and participated in multiple large prospective, multicenter studies. Since 2013 he is private professor at University of Szeged in Hungary.

Flanging 3-Piece IOLs

Shin Yamane

Abstract

The flanged intraocular lens (IOL) fixation technique is a minimally invasive way to fix IOLs in eyes without capsular support. The haptics of the IOL are externalized with two 30-gauge thin wall needles and heated to make flange. The flanges prevent the haptics falling off from the scleral tunnel. This technique is simple, but surgeons need to know some tips to make it successful. The positional relationships of the wounds, insertion angle of the needles, and grasping point of the haptics are important. The specific instruments are useful to improve the result.

Keywords

Flanged IOL fixation · Yamane technique · Dislocated IOL · Aphakia

Introduction

The flanged IOL fixation technique was developed to minimize surgical wounds and achieve firm haptic fixation without using suture or glue [1]. This technique is simple but not easy. There are some key points to make the surgery success.

Supplementary Information The online version contains supplementary material available at https://doi.org/10.1007/978-3-031-32855-8_3.

S. Yamane (✉)
Yamane Eye Clinic, 5-78-4F Aioi-Cho, Naka-Ku, Yokohama 235-0012, Kanagawa, Japan
e-mail: yamane.eyeclinic@gmail.com

Materials and Devices

1. Thirty-gauge thin wall needle; This needle (TSK Ultra Thin-Wall Needle) is available in Japan (Tochigi Seiko), US (Delasco Dermatologic Lab and Supply, Inc.), and Netherlands (TSK Laboratory Europe). The inner diameter of the needle must be 0.18 mm or more. Twenty-seven-gauge needles may also be used.
2. Ophthalmic cautery; Accu-Temp® Cautery (Beaver Visitec). Low temperature cautery is enough to make the flange on the tip of the haptic
3. Forceps; Special forceps for intrascleral IOL fixation (Yamane IOL fixation forceps (CVF4032-23 and CVO-HANDLE); Katalyst Surgical) are recommended. Other forceps for anterior segment surgery is available (e.g. Micro-Holding Forceps; MST). Long, straight forceps for vitreous surgery are not suitable, but disposable 25-G vitreoretinal forceps (eg, Grieshaber 25-G MaxiGrip forceps) can be used with gentle bending.
4. IOL; Most of 3-piece IOLs are available. However, an IOL with thick haptics that cannot be inserted into the needle is not available. Polyvinylidene difluoride (PVDF) is recommended as the material of the haptics. This material is hard to cause breakage or deformation during surgery due to its flexibility. The haptics of X-70 [Santen], PN6A [Kowa], and CT Lucia [Zeiss] are made of PVDF.
5. Needle stabilizer (Geuder); The needle stabilizer can hold eye ball and stabilize the insertion angle of the needles (Fig. 1) [2].

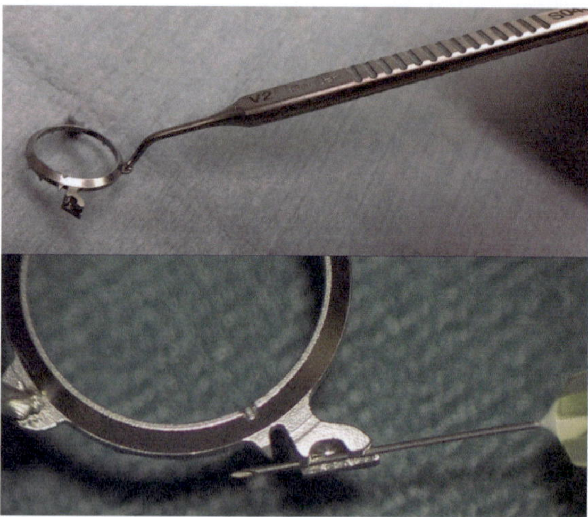

Fig. 1 The needle stabilizer has two wings with grooves for passing a needle on the outside of the ring-shaped body

Surgical Technique

1. Peripheral iridotomy using the vitrectomy cutter before mydriasis (Fig. 2).
2. Pars plana vitrectomy or anterior vitrectomy.
3. Subluxated crystalline lens or dislocated IOL removal.
4. A 3-piece IOL insertion into the anterior chamber. The trailing haptic must be kept outside the eye to prevent the IOL from falling into the vitreous cavity.
5. An angled sclerotomy made with a 30-gauge thin wall needle through the conjunctiva at 2.0–2.5 mm from the limbus (Fig. 3).

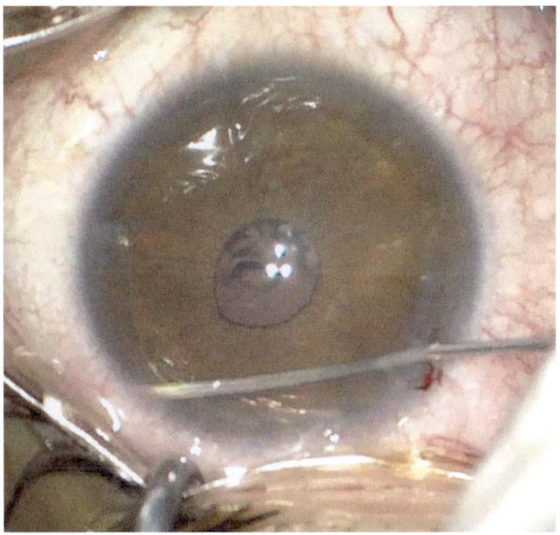

Fig. 2 Peripheral iridotomy was performed by a vitrectomy cutter

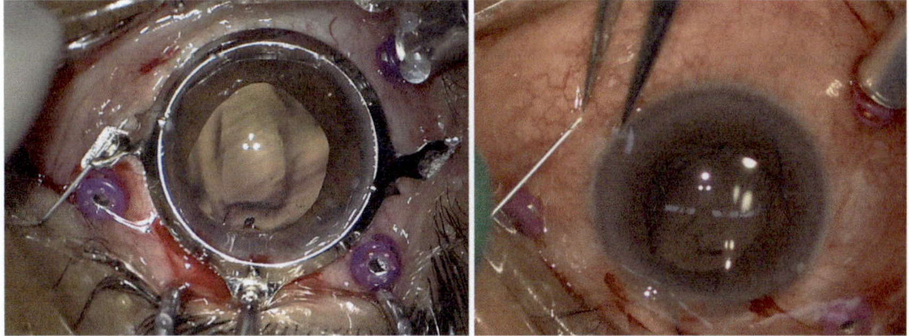

Fig. 3 Insertion of the 30-gauge thin wall needle with (left) and without (right) the needle stabilizer

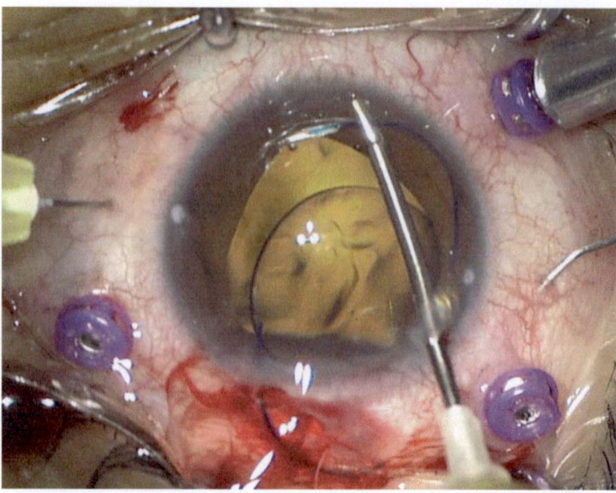

Fig. 4 Introduction of the leading haptic into the lumen of the 30-gauge needle

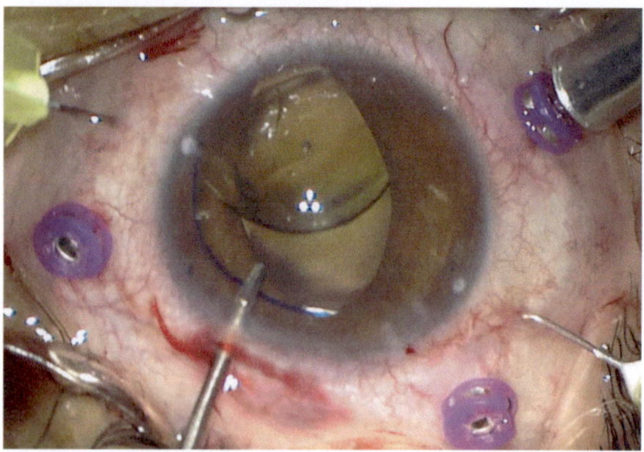

Fig. 5 Introduction of the trailing haptic into the lumen of the 30-gauge needle using the double-needle technique

6. Insertion of the leading haptic into the lumen of the needle using a forceps (Fig. 4). The needle that is not connected to a syringe is allowed to rest on the conjunctiva.
7. A second sclerotomy made with a 30-gauge thin wall needle at 180° from the first sclerotomy.
8. Insertion of the trailing haptic into the lumen of the second needle (double-needle technique: Fig. 5).
9. Externalization of the haptics onto the conjunctiva with the needles (Fig. 6).
10. Cauterization of the ends of the haptics using an ophthalmic cautery device to make a flange with a diameter of 0.3 mm (Fig. 7).
11. Fixation of the flange of the haptics into the scleral tunnels (Fig. 8).

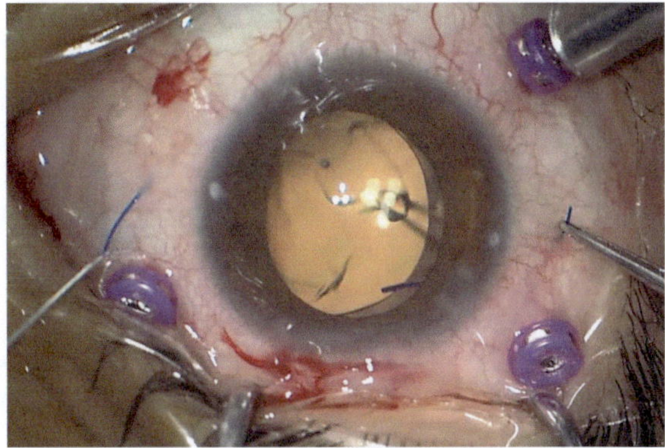

Fig. 6 Externalization of the haptics

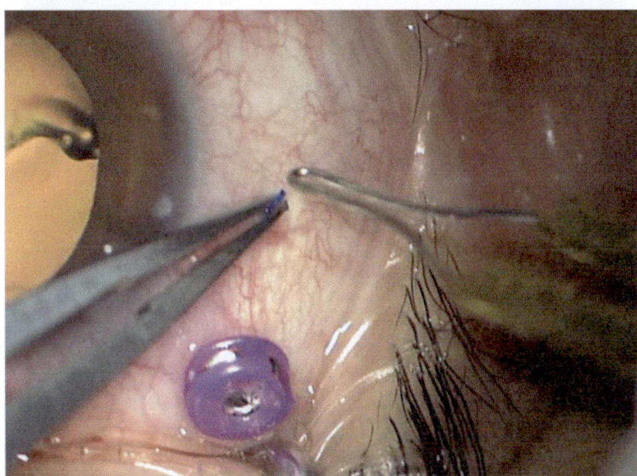

Fig. 7 Cauterization of the haptics to make flanges

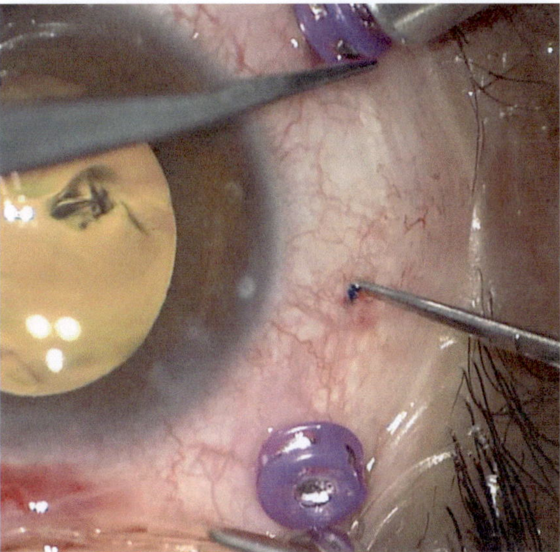

Fig. 8 Pushing back of the haptics to fix the flanges in the scleral tunnel

Results

Flanged IOL fixation was used on 150 eyes of 147 patients (103 men, 44 women; mean age 68.5 ± 13.3 years). Indications were IOL dislocation in 97 eyes, aphakia in 28 eyes, and the crystalline lens dislocation in 25 eyes. The mean corrected visual acuity was 0.30 logarithm of the minimum angle of resolution (logMAR) units preoperatively and 0.10, 0.10, 0.09, and 0.12 logMAR units at 3, 6, 12, and 24 months postoperatively. Four models of IOL were used in this series. The mean refractive difference from predicted value was −0.33D and the mean IOL tilt was 3.21° (Table 1). The most common postoperative complications was iris capture of IOL (5.3%). There was no severe complications, i.e., retinal detachment, endophthalmitis, and IOL dislocation (Table 2).

Table 1 Refractive difference from the predicted value

IOL model	Number	IOL power (D)	Refractive difference (mean ± SD, D)	IOL tilt (degree)
X-70 (Santen)	89	18.9 ± 4.0	−0.46 ± 0.97	3.32 ± 2.54
ZA9003 (Abbott Medical Optics)	32	17.9 ± 4.5	−0.02 ± 0.93	2.86 ± 2.18
PN6A (Kowa)	16	15.1 ± 7.9	−0.20 ± 0.86	2.56 ± 1.40
MA60MA (Alcon, Inc.)	6	−1.2 ± 4.5	0.95 ± 1.2	5.37 ± 3.58
Total	143	−17.3 ± 6.4	−0.33 ± 1.18	3.21 ± 2.44

SD standard deviation, *IOL* intraocular lens, *D* diopter

Table 2 Postoperative complications

Complications	Eyes, n (%)
Early complications	
Vitreous hemorrhage	5 (3.3%)
Hypotony	4 (2.7%)
IOP elevation	4 (2.7%)
Corneal edema	1 (0.7%)
Retinal tear	1 (0.7%)
Late complications	
Iris capture of IOL	8 (5.3%)
Cystoid macular edema	1 (0.7%)
IOP elevation	1 (0.7%)

IOP intraocular pressure

Complications and Countermeasures

Haptic deformation: IOL haptics can be bended or broken by grasping and pushing into needles hardly. The haptic and needle should be aligned before insertion to reduce inserting friction.

IOL decentration: IOL dislocation occurs when a scleral tunnel is not created 180° to the opposite side. In that case, one scleral tunnel should be recreated. If the IOL dislocation is seen despite the scleral tunnel is correctly formed, there is a possibility that the IOL haptic is deformed. In that case, the IOL should be exchanged.

IOL tilt: IOL tilt occurs when the angle of the scleral tunnel is not symmetrical. Especially, the angle in the vertical direction is easily deviated only by observation using a surgical microscope. The needle stabilizer is useful to control insertion angle of the needles. For eyes with a small corneal diameter, the flexure of the IOL haptics induce IOL tilt. In such cases, IOL tilt can be reduced by cutting the haptics before making flange.

Conclusions

The flanged IOL fixation technique is minimally invasive and provide firm haptic fixation. If mastered, good results can be obtained with a short time surgery. Proper wound positioning and the use of appropriate instruments for this surgery are the keys to success.

Acknowledgements Chapter reprinted with permission from Yamane, S. (2020). Secondary Intraocular Lens Implantation: Flanged IOL Fixation Techniques. In: Albert, D., Miller, J., Azar, D., Young, L.H. (eds) Albert and Jakobiec's Principles and Practice of Ophthalmology. Springer, Cham. https://doi.org/10.1007/978-3-319-90495-5_199-1.

Financial Support None.
Conflict of Interest No conflicting relationship exists for any author.

References

1. Yamane S, Sato S, Maruyama-Inoue M, Kadonosono K. Flanged intrascleral intraocular lens fixation with double-needle technique. Ophthalmology. 2017;124:1136–42.
2. Yamane S, Maruyama-Inoue M, Kadonosono K. Needle stabilizer for flanged intraocular lens fixation. Retina. 2019;39:801.

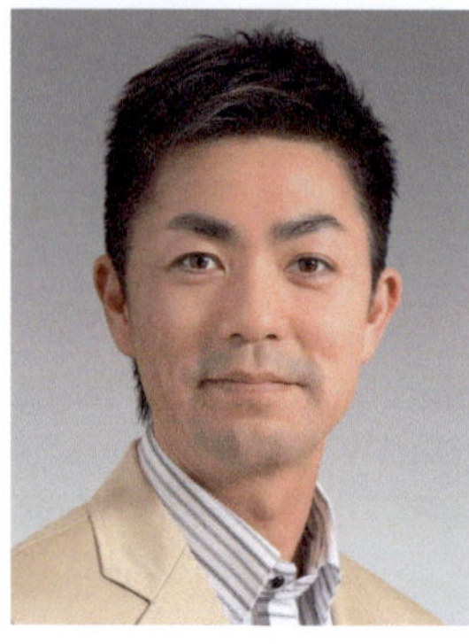

Shin Yamane graduated from Medical School in Yokohama City University in 2002. During his residency program he was trained in Yokohama City University Hospital and Yokohama City University Medical Center. From 2006 to 2009 he worked in Yokosuka Kyosai Hospital. In 2010, he became an assistant professor at the Yokohama City University Medical Center and in 2020 opened the Yamane Eye Clinic. Main focus in ophthalmic surgery are cataract and vitreoretinal surgery. He performs more than 2,000 surgeries per year. He has trained many surgeons and has been invited to many international conferences to give educational lectures. He has authored many scientific papers, published in Ophthalmology, AJO, Retina and others. He has won awards at international conferences such as ASCRS, ESCRS, and APACRS. The method of fixing the intraocular lens developed by him to the sclera is called the Yamane technique and is widely used all over the world. He himself successfully performed the Yamane technique at a live surgery at BRASCRS in 2019.

History and Evolution of Double Flanged Suture Fixation

Sérgio Canabrava

Abstract

The first use of polypropylene with flanges in ophthalmic surgery was presented in 2017 by Canabrava et al. in the American Society of Cataract and Refractive Surgery (ASCRS) Film Festival. The double-flanged polypropylene haptic, removed from a 3-piece Intraocular Lens (IOL), was initially used to fix Capsular Tension Segment (CTS) to the sclera and was described as a suture-free option with CTS for managing zonular weakness or dialysis of different etiologies in eyes undergoing cataract surgery.

Introduction

The first use of polypropylene with flanges in ophthalmic surgery was presented in 2017 by Canabrava et al. in the American Society of Cataract and Refractive Surgery (ASCRS) Film Festival. The double-flanged polypropylene haptic, removed from a 3-piece Intraocular Lens (IOL), was initially used to fix Capsular Tension Segment (CTS) to the sclera and was described as a suture-free option with CTS for managing zonular weakness or dialysis of different etiologies in eyes undergoing cataract surgery.

Supplementary Information The online version contains supplementary material available at https://doi.org/10.1007/978-3-031-32855-8_4.

S. Canabrava (✉)
Centro Oftalmológico de Minas Gerais, Belo Horizonte, MG, Brazil
e-mail: sergiocanabrava@hotmail.com

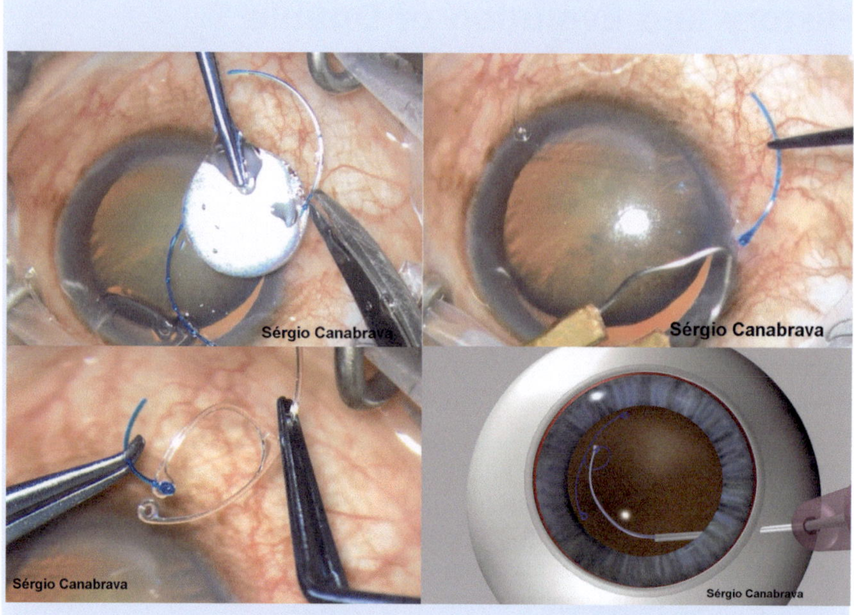

© Sergio Canabrava 2023. All Rights Reserved

This is a sequence of images from the first surgery with the Double Flanged Technique using a CTS to fixate a capsular bag. It was performed in 2016 and presented at the 2017 ASCRS Film Festival in San Diego. Note that the initial Double Flanged idea was inspired by the three-piece IOL used by Yamane for his scleral fixation technique. It was only in 2017 that we started our revolutionary research with Prolene thread

Later, in 2018, the technique was modified for our group and the haptic was replaced by 5-0 polypropylene suture and was applied in cases of subluxated cataracts and zonulopathies as Marfan syndrome. Using the versatility of the double flanged technique, our group published a new method for fixing non-foldable in 2019 naming it four-flanged technique.

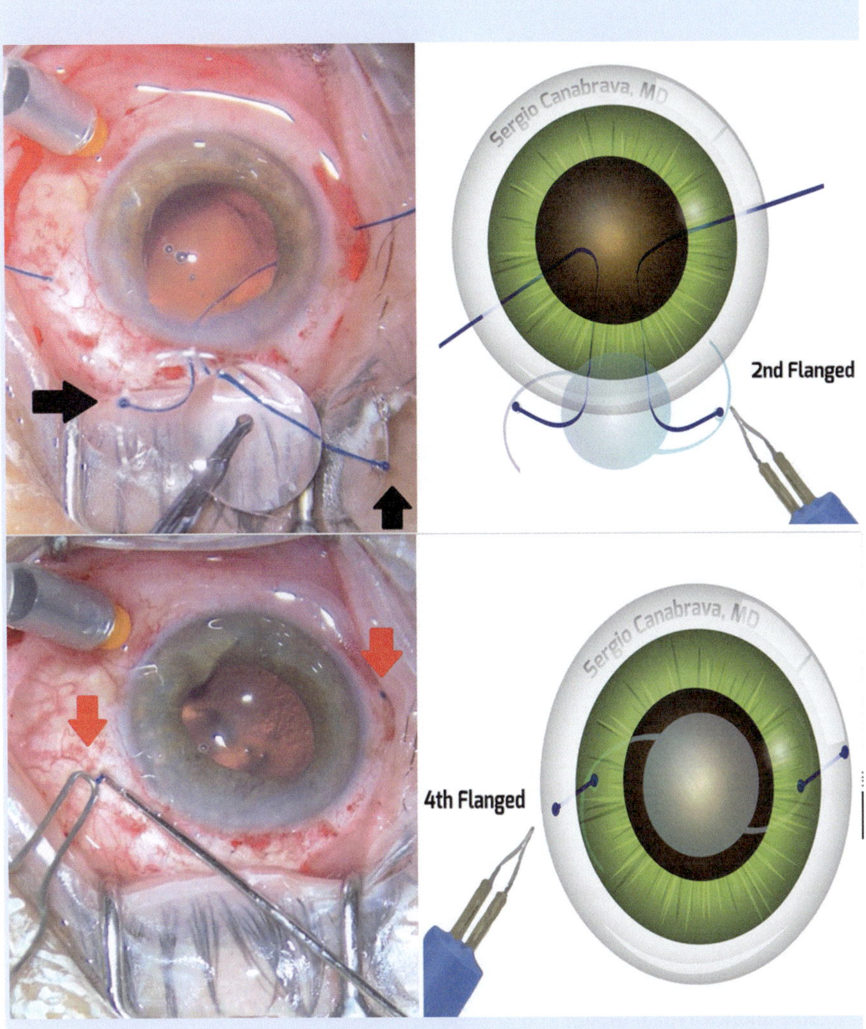

In these images we can observe the use of the Polypropylene to fixate a Non-Foldable IOL in the sclera. After proving that the use of double flanged polypropylene was effective for CTS, this was the second use presented by our group for the technique

Later in 2019, our group presented our third use of the Double Flanged, fixating an 4 loops foldable IOL in the scleral.

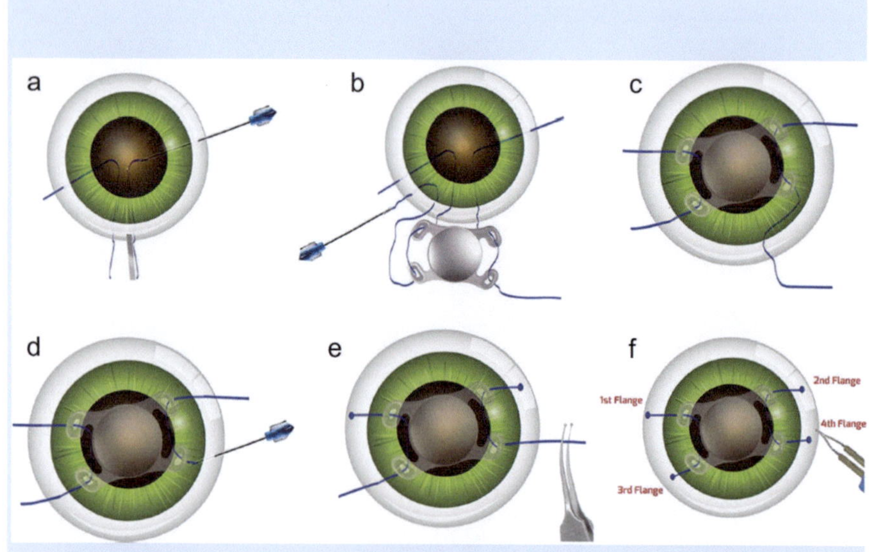

We can observe the steps to fixate a 4 Loops Foldable IOL in the Scleral using the Double Flanged Polypropylene Technique

Double Flanged Technique with Others Authors

Later on, new uses for the technique were published in the scientific literature. Being versatile, it allowed for other applications such as repairing iridodialysis (Kusaka M from Japan), piercing IOLs (Durval Jr, from Brazil), repositioning of subluxated IOLs in a variety of intraocular lenses as hydrophilic, hydrophobic, and polymethyl methacrylate aniridic IOLs (Altan Atakan, from Turkey) and the capsular anchor (AssiAnchor).

With five years already passed after performing the double-flanged technique in many eyes, we had the opportunity to assess the long-term outcomes of this technique.

In this chapter, we will present our experience with the Double Flanged Technique and evaluated the double-flanged technique for long-term stability of the flanges as well as possible late complications and surgical mistakes that can cause them.

Complications in the Technique

When we wrote this chapter, we had 71 eyes followed and 5 years of technique. Overall, 71 eyes of 61 patients were evaluated. The mean follow-up period for these eyes was 28.2 months. 173 flanges were performed. Thirteen cases with sub-Tenon flanges (7.5%) were observed. Five exposed flanges (2.89%) presented after a mean of 1.8 weeks postoperatively were observed. One patient with large flange presented with conjunctival inflammation and hyperemia. Two late internalized flanges (1.1%) and 2 recently internalized flanged (1.1%) were observed. Three eyes (4.22%) had retinal detachment. Also, cystoid macular edema was detected in 3 eyes (4.22%). No cases of endophthalmitis we observed.

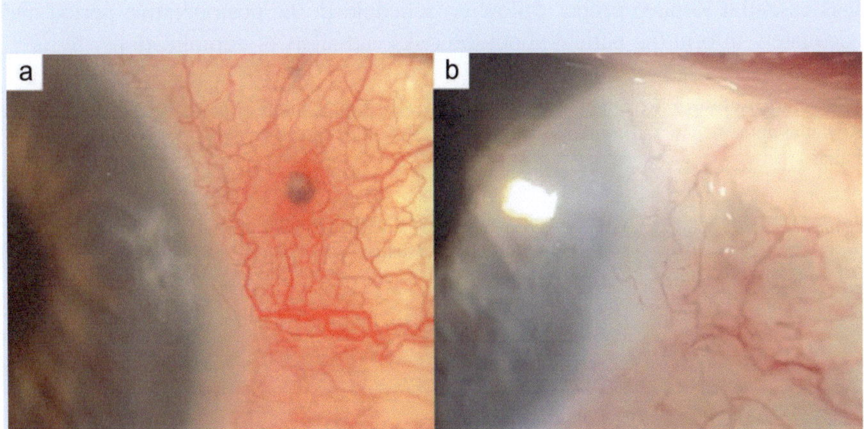

The flange outside the scleral tunnel with hyperemia and conjunctival inflammation and degradation (A). No conjunctival degradation or hyperemia after surgical reduction of the flange and reinsertion in the scleral tunnel (B). This was due to a very large flanged and outside the scleral tunnel

Tips to Avoid Complication in the Technique

After many years researching the double flanged technique, we suggest some tips to avoid complications with the technique: (1) careful choice of the material used: for 5-0 polypropylene, the best needle is the 27G insulin needle, whereas 6-0 polypropylene suture requires 29G insulin needle; (2) mark 2 mm from the limbus; (3) create a long scleral tunnel that is parallel to the limbus and about 2 mm long; (4) increase the tension of the polypropylene suture by holding its base with the 23-gauge micro forceps in close apposition to the sclera; (5) the polypropylene suture should be cut 1.2–1.5 mm from the micro forceps; (6) dry the prolene and do not touch it with the thermocautery when to make the flanged; (7) make sure that the flange is completely buried within the scleral tunnel at the end of the surgery; (8) be careful when piercing the IOL. After several trials, some patients were found to have tilted IOL, so, we discontinued this technique.

Conclusion

The many years follow-up of cases that underwent double-flanged technique shows that the technique is safe and effective if the right steps are taken. The surgeon should bear in mind that each flange is at risk of erosion or exposition, so at the end of the surgery, they would better make sure that the flange is properly buried. It is essential to have proper follow-up schedule in the postoperative period and adequately inform the patient about the risks and signs of complications.

Financial Disclosure Royalties agreement with AJL Ophthalmic—Spain to Canabrava Ring. Royalties agreement with Bioniko Models—USA. Royalties agreement with Madhu Instruments—India.

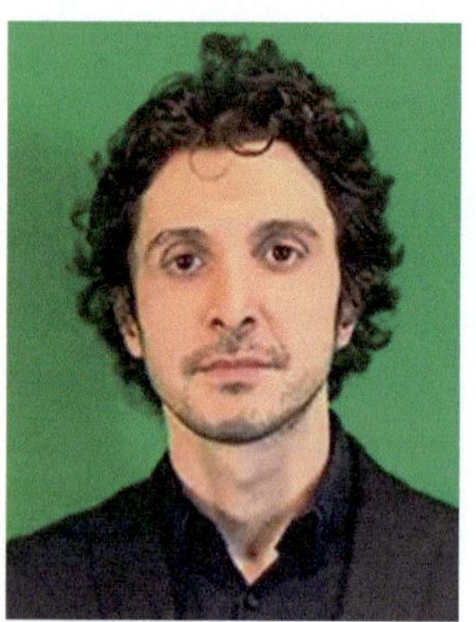

Sérgio Canabrava Centro Oftalmológico de Minas Gerais, Belo Horizonte, MG, Brazil.

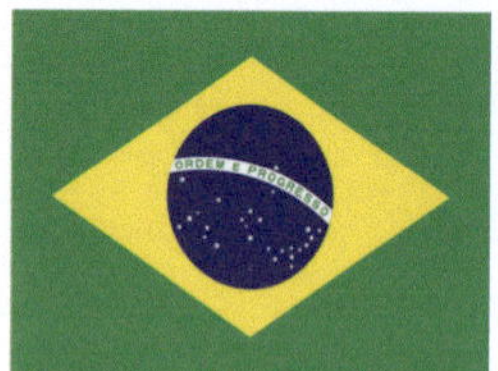

Flanging Intraocular Lenses and Devices in Special Situations

Avner Belkin and Ehud I. Assia

Abstract

This chapter describes the multitude of uses for flanged scleral fixation in anterior segment surgery and sets the stage for further innovations. The flange technique can be effectively utilized in cases of aphakia, subluxated or dislocated lenses inside or outside of the capsular bag, and for the fixation of anterior segment implants and devices. Surgical decision making is addressed, specific techniques are detailed, and pearls for success are discussed.

Keywords

Capsular stabilizing devices · Zonular support · Scleral fixation · IOL subluxation · Flange fixation

Introduction

Flanging is a major development in anterior segment surgery. A mark of a lasting and impactful advancement is its ability to inspire further innovations, and to be applicable in a diverse range of clinical scenarios. Shin Yamane pioneered flanging of intraocular lens (IOL) haptics [1]. Though this technique is definitely a landmark innovation in anterior segment surgery and has gained worldwide popularity, it is limited to 3-piece lenses. Sergio Canabrava extended the flanging principles by using non-integrated polypropylene sutures [2], thus expanding its use to a large

Supplementary Information The online version contains supplementary material available at https://doi.org/10.1007/978-3-031-32855-8_5.

A. Belkin · E. I. Assia (✉)
Department of Ophthalmology, Meir Medical Center, Kfar Saba, Israel
e-mail: Assia@eintal.com

Ein Tal Eye Center, Tel-Aviv, Israel

variety of IOLs and capsule stabilizing devices [3]. There are numerous applications for flanging in anterior segment surgery, and this technique tends to be especially useful in special cases, some of which will be covered in this chapter.

Flanged Fixation of IOLs in Aphakia with No Capsular Support

The use of flanged IOL haptics [1] for primary or secondary implantation of a scleral fixated IOL in cases of aphakia has gained widespread popularity since the initial reports by Yamane. A 3-piece IOL is inserted into the anterior chamber, the haptics are externalized through 27–30G needles and the tips of the haptic are heated using cautery to create a wide flange acting like the head of a nail. This technique requires high skills and experience and is associated with numerous complications such as haptic detachment, IOL drop and dislocation, lens tilt and others. Using separate 5-0 polypropylene sutures, as suggested by Canabrava, allows passing the sutures through the scleral wall prior to insertion of the IOL, making this technique significantly safer and more predictable with less intraocular manipulations. The lenses used for this purpose included IOLs with 2–4 eyelets (usually hard PMMA lenses) or closed-loop haptics (foldable acrylic lenses). Assia and Wong suggested using a 6-0 polypropylene suture for its tendency to be less stiff and more "user friendly" than the 5-0 suture (3). Recently, 7-0 prolene suture has been suggested for fixation, though some surgeons find these sutures to be less comfortable and too soft to serve as "pseudo-haptics". Two-point fixation of PC-IOLs can be associated with lens decentration and IOL tilt leading to significant optical aberrations. A popular lens design for secondary IOL implantation in aphakia with no capsular support using flanged sutures is the 4-closed-loop haptic design [4]. The sutures can be inserted transsclerally and then externalized through the main incision and threaded through the nostril of the cartridge prior to lens injection into the anterior chamber. This may cause confusion due to criss-crossing of the multiple sutures present in the anterior chamber during IOL insertion. Alternatively, the IOL can first be inserted into the anterior chamber and the suture fixation is done when the IOL is already inside the eye.

Even though 4 closed-loop haptics provide a stable and predictable fixation, if the loops are wide and soft, they can override each other when tightening the sutures, making control over final placement difficult. We have recently modified a plate-haptic PC-IOL with 4 holes giving the surgeon easier, more direct control over IOL position. Also, since control over the fixation axis is determined by suture location, and the lens cannot rotate parallel to the iris, implanting toric plate haptic IOLs using suture flanged fixation is an attractive option. Initial clinical experience is excellent making this lens design ideal for its purpose (unpublished data) (Fig. 1).

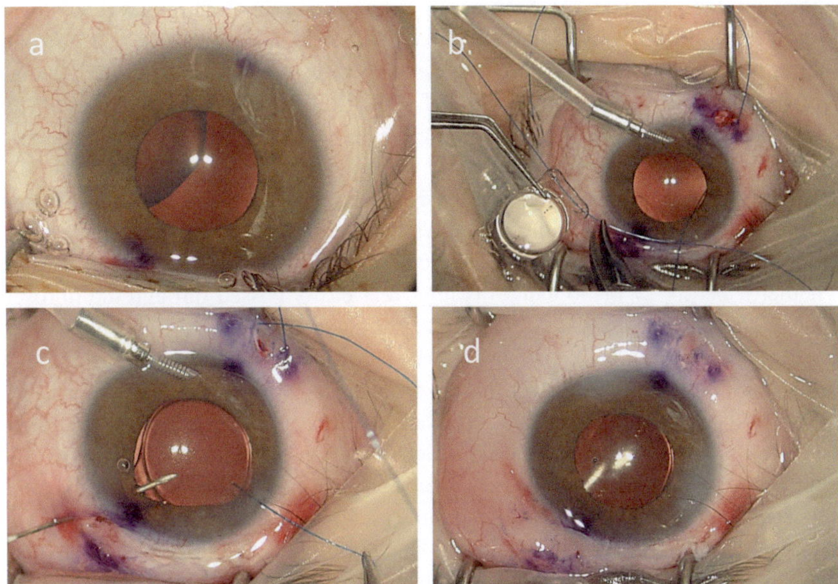

Fig. 1 Secondary implantation of a plate haptic toric IOL. A subluxated crystalline lens, with the axis marked for implantation (a). After lens removal, a 6-0 polypropylene suture is threaded through two islets of the plate-haptic IOL, and are externalized through the sclera (b). The IOL is inserted into the posterior chamber, and the sutures are threaded into the remaining two islets (c). At the end of surgery the IOL is well centered, at the planned axis (d)

Flanged Fixation of Subluxated IOLs

In cases in which an IOL is subluxated, repositioning and fixation of the same IOL is a good alternative to IOL exchange. The advantages of repositioning over exchange (providing the current IOL is of satisfactory optical quality) are less manipulations in the anterior chamber with increased endothelial safety, smaller incisions, and simpler surgery. Techniques to reposition and scleral fixate have been known for over 30 years [5–7]. Introduction of flanging techniques has allowed for further innovations in this space [8, 9] making surgical correction of this increasingly common phenomena more approachable to the anterior segment surgeon.

Prior to beginning the refixation surgery, a focused assessment of the anterior segment is warranted. First, the amount and extent of zonular weakness should be addressed. Cases with diffuse widespread lack of zonular support tend to be more prone to post-operative IOL tilt. If there is an area with intact zonules, surgery should proceed in a manner that preserves this area by minimizing traction in the opposite direction. Second, it is important to note the relationship of the IOL to the capsular bag. This includes whether the lens is completely in the bag, the overlap of the anterior capsulorhexis over the lens optic, the shape and position of the haptics and the presence of a Sommering's ring. The two main reasons to address a Sommering's ring during IOL re-fixation are its potential to push the IOL forward leading to friction on the posterior iris and causing Uveitis Glaucoma Hyphema (UGH) syndrome, and the possibility of IOL tilt. The Sommering's ring can be removed by aspiration or by maneuvering the lens material out of the capsular bag and removing it by phacoemulsification or anterior vitrectomy. In terms of IOL design: If the IOL has an open-loop design, it is recommended that the IOL-bag complex be suture-fixated to the scleral wall as one unit. This minimizes the risk of suture slippage and adds stability. The needle used as a guide for flanged fixation (whether it be 26, 27 or 30 gauge) is relatively easily passed through the fibrosed capsule surrounding the haptic to achieve this goal. If the IOL is of closed loop design, it can be fixated also if it is located outside of the capsular bag through the closed haptic loops.

The basic steps of flange fixation using 6-0 prolene and a 30G needle have been previously described [8, 9]. After lens position in the anterior chamber has been thoroughly assessed as outlined above, the limbus is marked at two points 180° apart. The markings need to take into consideration current and planned IOL position. The edge of a 6-0 prolene is cut in an oblique fashion to create a diagonal edge and inserted into the anterior chamber through a paracentesis. The free edge is docked into a 30G bent needle that has been inserted through the sclera 1.5–2.0 mm behind the limbus, under the haptic and through the capsule close to the optic haptic junction. The suture is then externalized through the sclera and a temporary flange using thermo-cautery is created. The maneuver is repeated with the second edge of the suture, this time passing the needle above the haptic. The suture thus engulfs the haptic and the fibrosed capsule, preventing slippage. This procedure is then repeated on the opposite side. The tension of the suture is adjusted by repeated diathermy until the lens is central and stable. Tension adjustment is one more advantage of the flanging technique, in contrast to other suturing techniques in which suture tension cannot be changed once a knot is locked (Fig. 2).

For in-the-bag fixation of open-loop IOLs, we recommend positioning the two flanged suture ends radial (1 and 2 mm from the limbus on the same meridian), as opposed to parallel to the limbus. This prevents the torque on the haptics thus decreasing the risk of IOL tilt [8].

Alternatives to Optic-Haptic Junction Fixation

A suture around the haptic may not be sufficient for stable IOL fixation, for example, in eyes in which the haptic is located outside of the capsular bag. Nevertheless, even in these cases flanged scleral fixation is still often possible using alternative techniques. Canabrava suggested creating a small round hole in the lens using a designated proprietary punch [10]. Micheletti designed an intraocular micro-punch for lenses already located inside the eye (not yet commercially available).

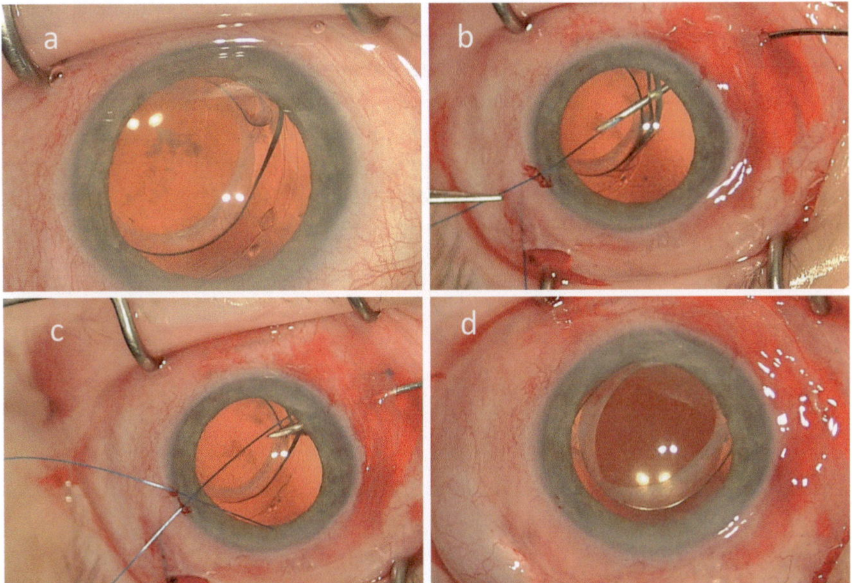

Fig. 2 Flanged scleral fixation of a subluxated IOL. A subluxated in-the-bag foldable acrylic IOL (a). A 30G needle is passed 2 mm from the limbus and into the posterior chamber under the haptic, through the capsule, close to the optic-haptic junction. The 6-0 prolene is inserted into the lumen of the needle (b). The needle is inserted 1 mm anterior to the previous insertion point, this time passing above the haptic (c). The IOL is centered and stable at the end of surgery (d)

Assia et al. suggested direct fixation of soft lenses by penetrating the lens material either by the needle of the 6-0 prolene suture, or by using a 30G needle serving as a guide for the prolene suture (3). They showed that the needle can penetrate any type of soft IOL (hydrophobic, hydrophilic or silicone), at any location (optic or haptic), preferably at the optic-haptic junction (Fig. 3). This expands the IOL choice to practically any foldable lens since holes or closed loops are not mandatory. After the suture passes through the lens material a flange is created and pulled into the eye until it contacts the IOL to create an "internal flange". It is preferable to pass the needle from the back surface of the IOL to the anterior surface so the internal flange will be located behind (posterior) to the optic and would not cause chaffing of the iris and pigment dispersion. The flange should be relatively wide, and the surgeon should be very careful not to exert tension on the suture as it may cheese-wire through the lens material. One major advantage of this technique is that it can be used to fixate IOLs already located inside the eye (8) (Fig. 4). Since suture location is not dependent on existing holes or closed loops the needle pass can be located at any part of the lens. A 3- or 4-point fixation may provide more stability to the IOL, compensate for decentration at any direction or correct IOL tilt (Fig. 5). Passing a needle through the lens material can be challenging, and can cause stress on the remaining zonules or drag the IOL while pulling the suture because of friction forces. It is important to use a second-hand instrument to provide counter-pressure such as a hook or microforceps to hold the IOL steady. In special cases the surgeon may also utilize remaining fibrosed capsule and suture it directly to the scleral wall without passing through the IOL material. The guiding 30G needle is passed through the capsulorhexis, between the capsule and the IOL optic, penetrating the capsule as close as possible to the capsular equator, and externalized after penetrating the scleral wall. The second half of the prolene suture is threaded through the needle passing in front of the lens capsule (Fig. 6).

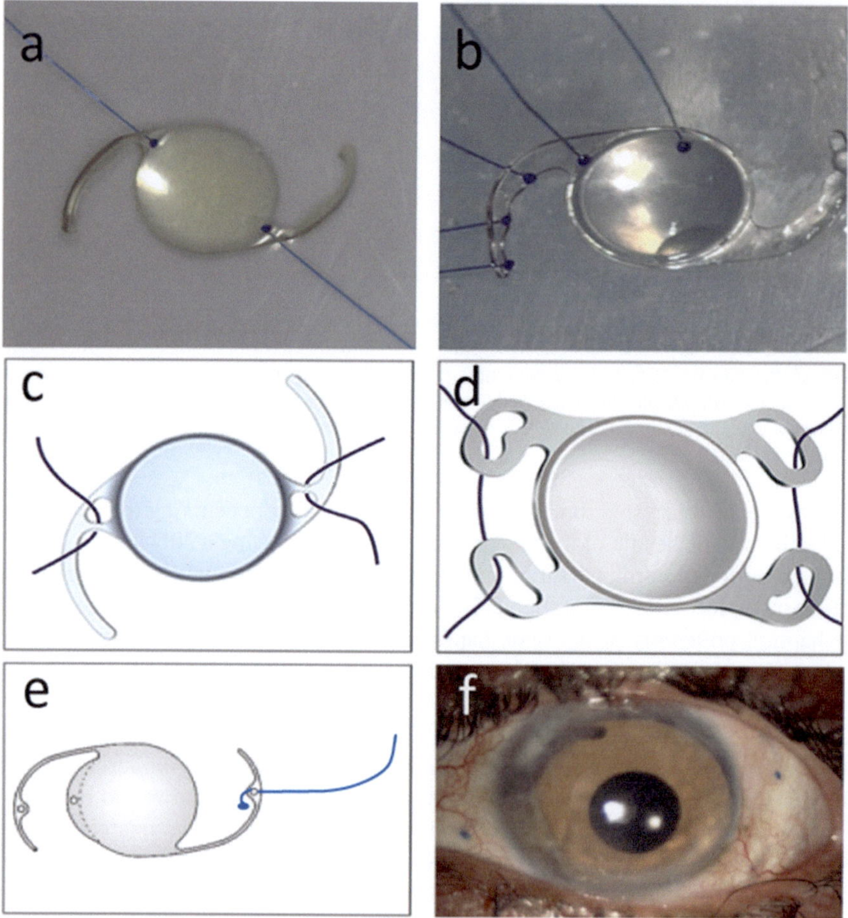

Fig. 3 Flanging in different materials and locations. Two-point fixation in a hydrophobic lens (a), multiple flanges in a hydrophilic lens in the optic, junction, and along the haptic in a laboratory model (b), two point fixation through the islet in a hydrophobic lens (c), 4 point fixation in a 4-haptic IOL design (d), two-point fixation through haptic islets in a PMMA IOL (e), and flange fixation of an aniridic prosthesis (f)

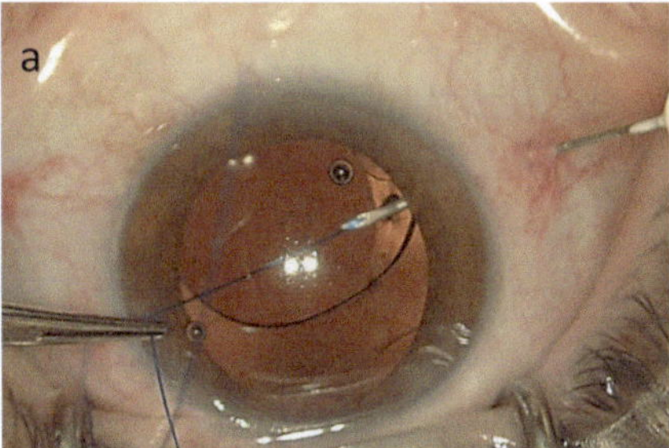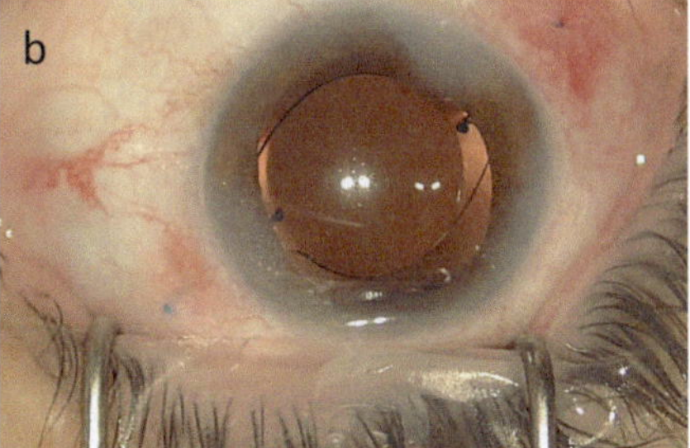

Fig. 4 Flange fixation through IOL material. A 30G needle is passed through the lens material at the optic-haptic junction and the 6-0 prolene is threaded through it (a). At the end of surgery, the lens is centered and stable, with the internal flanges located anterior to the lens (b)

Fig. 5 Centration of scleral fixated IOL. After initial flanged fixation (black arrows) the IOL was decentered horizontally. A third trans-optic flange (white arrow) was used to center the lens

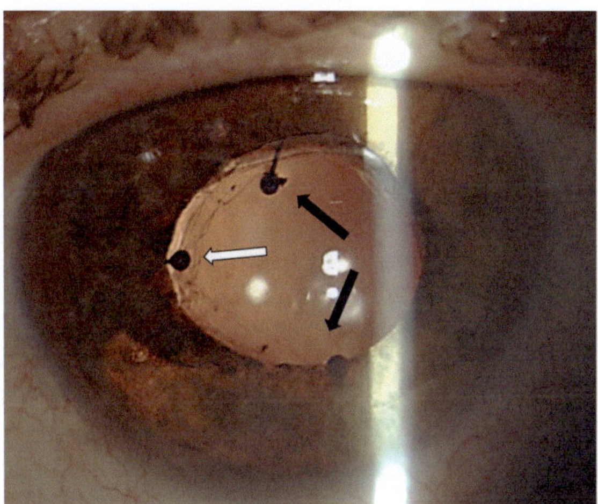

Fixating Capsular Tension Rings or Capsule Stabilizing Devices

Suture fixation of a malpositioned capsular bag containing a preplaced capsular tension ring (CTR) can be performed using a variety of sutures, the most common being 9-0, 10-0 polypropylene, or 7-0 Gore-Tex. While the thin (10-0 and 9-0) prolene sutures run the risk of suture degradation over time, the Gore-Tex suture is not intended for intraocular use, its needle is not designed for working inside the eye, and its use is off label. Flanged suture fixation is exceptionally suited for these cases for several reasons. Flanged sutures provide an easily titratable tension and the 6-0 prolene is sturdy and will not degrade over time. Also, knots of sutures must be buried inside the scleral tissue otherwise they may extrude through the conjunctiva whereas the rounded flanges can be covered by the conjunctiva and tenon with low risk of extrusion even years after surgery. Capsular tension rings

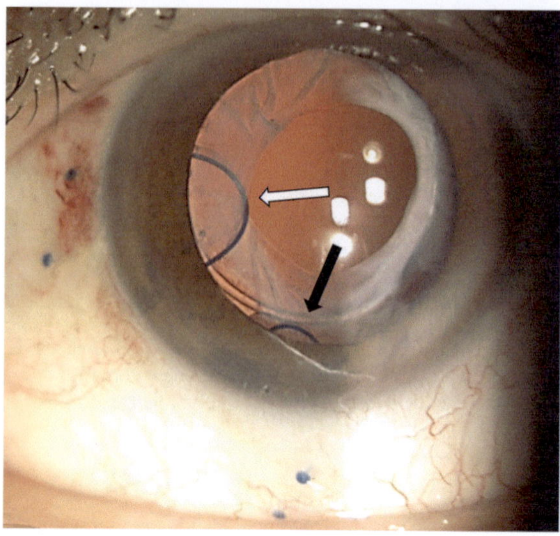

Fig. 6 Centration of scleral fixated IOL. After initial flanged fixation (black arrow) the IOL was decentered horizontally. A third loop was created around the fibrosed anterior capsule (white arrow) to center the lens

can be sutured to the scleral wall at any location, unrelated to the haptic axis and multiple-point fixation can be created.

In eyes with weak or missing zonules the capsular bag can still be utilized to maintain and fixate the IOL by suturing capsule stabilizing devices to the scleral wall. The modified Cionni ring and its modifications the Ahmed Segment and the Malyugin-Cionni ring are the most popular devices. Canabrava was the first to describe flanged fixation of a capsular tension ring or segment [11] to the sclera, using a 5-0 polypropylene suture to achieve the same goal (A). Assia described stabilizing the capsular bag to the scleral wall using the capsular Anchor (AssiAnchor, Hanita Lenses, Israel) with the 6-0 polypropylene suture and the adjustable flange technique (3) (Fig. 7). A second generation of the Anchor was recently developed to facilitate simpler surgery and has proven efficacious in cases of both subluxated crystalline and synthetic IOLs (12). The basic surgical steps for fixating the capsular Anchor are similar to those of suturing CTRs with fixating elements or capsular tension segments of different kinds. A 30G bent needle is inserted 2 mm from the limbus at the zone of the zonular weakness. A 6-0 prolene suture is inserted into the eye through a paracentesis or the main incision and docked into the needle, which is removed from the eye. The other end of the 6-0 prolene suture is externalized through the main incision. Outside of the eye the suture is threaded into the hole at the edge of the central rod of the Anchor, and a flange is created. Care must be taken that the flange is larger than the diameter of the hole and that it is located at the posterior face of the Anchor to reduce the risk of iris chaffing. The Anchor is inserted into the eye and maneuvered into place on the capsule edge with the central rod anterior to the capsule and the two lateral prongs posterior to it, inside the capsular bag. The Anchor is pulled peripherally using the externalized suture, with the rounded edges of the side prongs positioned against the equator. The suture is shortened with the Anchor in place. A small amount of

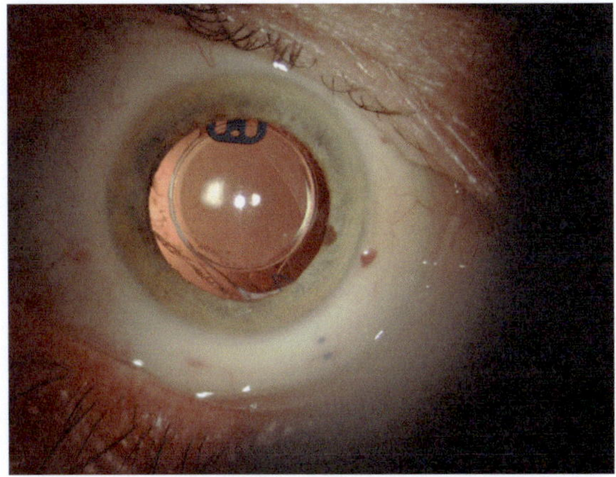

Fig. 7 Two point flange fixation to the scleral wall. The bottom fixation is done by passing a 6-0 prolene loop through the islet in the IOL haptic, and the superior fixation is done by using a first generation AssiaAnchor which holds the anterior capsule

suture should remain to allow for final adjustments at the end of surgery after IOL implantation to ascertain lens centration (Fig. 8). A similar technique was successfully used to refixate subluxated IOLs by creation pockets between the lens capsule and the IOL to allow insertion of the capsular Anchor.

In summary: primary or secondary fixation of intraocular lenses with no capsular support, refixation of malpositioned lenses and securing the capsular bag using capsule stabilizing devices can all be effectively done utilizing a variety of surgical flanging techniques.

Key Takeaways

1. Flanging techniques have made lens fixation surgery readily accessible to the anterior segment surgeon.
2. Flanging can be utilized in numerous surgical scenarios, and are an effective intra-operative problem solving tool.

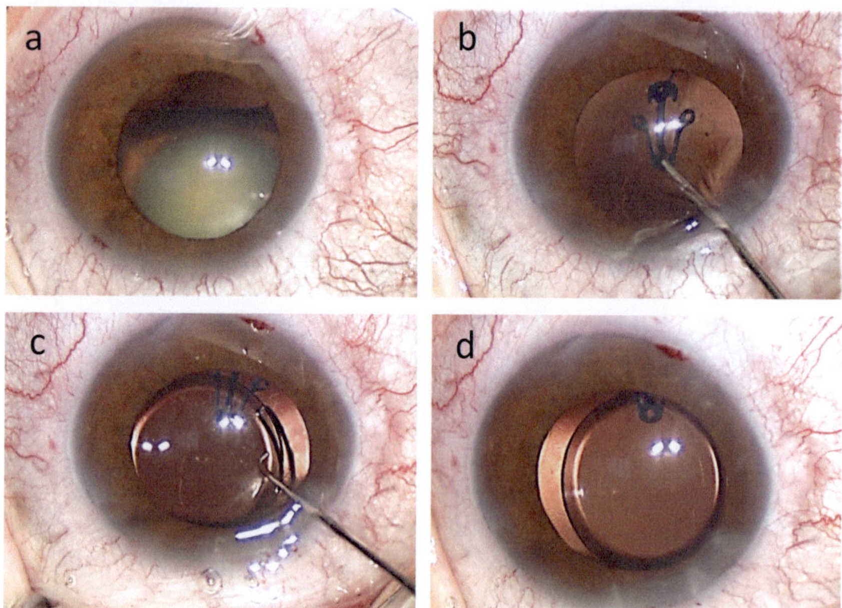

Fig. 8 Fixation of the capsular bag to the scleral wall using the second generation AssiaAnchor. A subluxated crystalline lens (a). After cataract removal, the Anchor is placed inside the capsular bag, with the cental rod above the anterior capsule and the two side prongs beneath it (b). An IOL is inserted (c), and the capsular bag is centered by titrating the suture at the flange by using diathermy (d)

References

1. Yamane S, et al. Flanged intrascleral intraocular lens fixation with double-needle technique. Ophthalmology. 2017;124(8):1136–42.
2. Canabrava S, Lima ACCD, Ribeiro G. Four-flanged intrascleral intraocular lens fixation technique: no flaps, no knots, no glue. Cornea. 2020;39(4):527–8.
3. Assia EI, Wong JXH. Adjustable 6-0 polypropylene flanged technique for intrascleral lens fixation. Part 1: primary fixation of intraocular lens in aphakia, fixation of capsular stabilizing devices, and fixation of aniridia implant. J Cat Refract Surge 2020;46:1387–91.
4. Mahler OS, et al. Modification of intraocular lens insertion using 4-flanged fixation with a standard cartridge and a 2.4 mm corneal incision in eyes with no capsular support. J Cataract Refract Surg. 2021;47(9):1227–33.
5. Azar DT, Wiley WF. Double-knot transscleral suture fixation technique for displaced intraocular lenses. Am J Ophthalmol. 1999;128(5):644–6.
6. Bloom SM, Wyszynski RE, Brucker AJ. Scleral fixation suture for dislocated posterior chamber intraocular lens. Ophthalmic Surg. 1990;21(12):851–4.
7. Chan CK. An improved technique for management of dislocated posterior chamber implants. Ophthalmology. 1992;99(1):51–7.
8. Assia EI, Wong JXH. Adjustable 6–0 polypropylene flanged technique for scleral fixation, part 2: repositioning of subluxated IOLs. J Cataract Refract Surg. 2020;46(10):1392–6.

9. Mahler OS, et al. Intrascleral 4-flanged technique for in-the-bag intraocular lens subluxation. J Cataract Refract Surg. 2021;47(4):476–81.
10. Canabrava S. 4-Flanged technique with a foldable IOL. 2019 [cited 21 Jan 2023; Video]. Available from: https://www.aao.org/clinical-video/4-flanged-technique-with-foldable-iol.
11. Canabrava S, et al. Double-flanged-haptic and capsular tension ring or segment for sutureless fixation in zonular instability. Int Ophthalmol. 2018;38(6):2653–62.
12. Belkin A, Yehezkeli V, Assia EI. The 2nd generation capsular anchor for subluxated lenses—first clinical results. J Cataract Refract Surg. 2022;48:564–7.
13. Canabrava S. Double flanged technique. Video J Catataract Refract Glaucoma Surg. Available at: https://vjcrgs.com/volume35-issue1/double-flanged-technique. Accessed 20 Dec 2022.

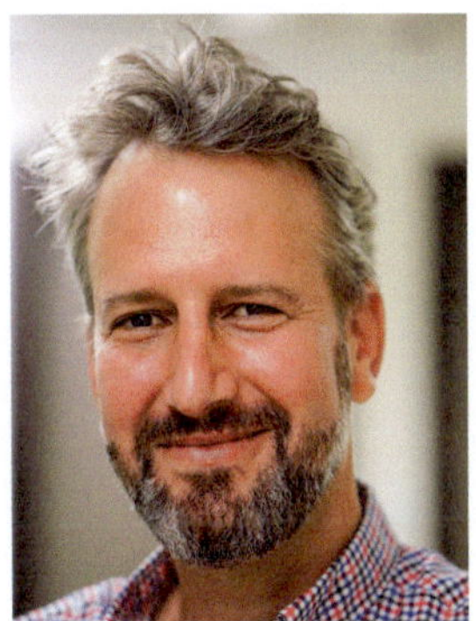

Avner Belkin graduated the Joyce and Irving Goldman Medical School in 2009. He completed his residency in Ophthalmology at the Meir Medical Center. He graduated from two fellowships: one in comprehensive adult Glaucoma and one in Glaucoma and advanced anterior segment surgery, both at the University of Toronto, Canada. Dr. Belkin is the director of the Glaucoma service at the Meir Medical Center, and a senior lecturer at the Sackler school of medicine at the Tel-Aviv University.

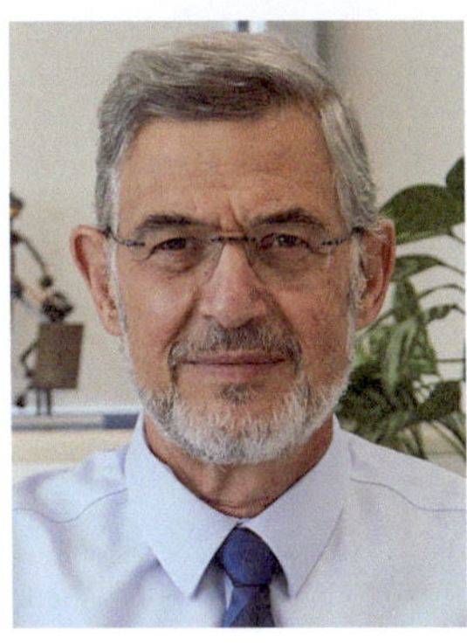

Ehud I. Assia graduated the Sackler School of Medicine at the Tel-Aviv University in 1980 (Magna Cum Laude) and has a Master degree in Ophthalmology (Summa Cum Laude, 1989). He did his residency in Ophthalmology at the Goldschleger Eye Institute, Sheba Medical Center, Israel. He completed research fellowship at the Center for Intraocular Lens Research at the Medical University of South Carolina, Charleston, SC, USA. Dr. Assia was the Director of the Department of Ophthalmology at the Meir Medical Center, Kfar-Saba, between 1994–2018 and was the Director of the Center for Applied Eye Research there in 2018–2022. Dr Assia is Full Professor at the Tel-Aviv University and was the Director of the Department of Ophthalmology of the Sackler School of Medicine between 1998–2002. He published over 200 peer-reviewed papers, 35 chapters in books, and over 50 additional publications. He is a co-author of a book on "Premium and specialized Intraocular lenses". He was the Chief Editor of the Israeli Journal of Eye Update for 23 years. Dr Assia developed several original patented devices and instruments for cataract and glaucoma surgery, accommodative IOL and more. Prof. Assia delivered several named lectures including the Lim Lecture (APACRS, 2012) and the Binkhorst Lecture (ESCRS, 2019) and received lifetime awards including the Senior Achievement Award of the American Academy of Ophthalmology (AAO, 2020). He is the Medical Director of the Ein Tal Eye Center, and the Ein Tal–Hadassah Laser Refractive Center in Tel-Aviv, Israel.

Decision-Making: IOL Refixation, IOL Exchange and Correction of Aphakia

Michael Amon, Wolfgang Geitzenauer, and Konstantin Seiller-Tarbuk

Abstract

This chapter describes the numerous options when treating IOL dislocation or aphakia. A systematic approach will guide the surgeon through the decision making process in different situations of IOL dislocation, IOL intolerance or aphakia. Different techniques of refixation and exchange of IOLs as well as options for IOL selection will be described. In addition, figures and videos will highlight each surgical step. By selective description of individual cases arguments for the best choice of the surgical technique and the implant will be created. Care will be taken to find the most suitable and least traumatic technique for each specific situation. Arguments and factors for IOL refixation or for IOL exchange are collected. Pros and cons of each technique will be discussed and guidance for the choice of the most suitable implant and surgical technique is given.

Keywords

Intraocular lens dislocation · IOL fixation · IOL refixation · IOL exchange · Yamane technique · Canabrava technique · Amon forceps-needle · Aphakia · Aniridia · Capsular tension ring · Flanging · Haptic · Suture

Supplementary Information The online version contains supplementary material available at https://doi.org/10.1007/978-3-031-32855-8_6.

M. Amon (✉) · W. Geitzenauer · K. Seiller-Tarbuk
Academic Teaching Hospital of St. John Vienna, Sigmund Freud Medical University, Vienna, Austria
e-mail: amon@augenchirurg.com

Introduction

IOL dislocation, IOL damage, IOL intolerance and aphakia:

Late onset of IOL subluxation or luxation is increasing significantly over the years [1–4]. One cause of this complication is the increase in life expectancy and the fact that our surgical technique has made progress and become significantly more precise. We perform cataract surgery and lens implantation more and more atraumatic. Hence, we continue to save more capsular bags for proper IOL implantation compared to the decades before. Especially in eyes with pseudoexfoliation it has been shown that the incidence of late IOL dislocation is significantly higher compared to standard eyes. The mean time from surgery to clinically significant dislocation is 6.9 to 8.5 years [4, 5]. But not only pseudoexfoliation is correlated with IOL dislocation: genetic diseases resulting in a lack of sufficient zonular support (such as Marfan syndrome or Marchesani syndrome), high myopia, trauma or metabolic diseases may also cause this complication [6–8].

Some patients present with a sudden dislocation of the IOL. Causes might be previous or current eye trauma or intraoperative complications such as severe zonular defects. An inadvertent damage of the IOL haptic or IOL optic might force us to even exchange the whole IOL already intraoperatively.

Opacified and damaged optics have to be exchanged either. Especially implants with multifocal optics are susceptible to decentration and may urge us to IOL exchange in case of lack of neuroadaptation or photic phenomena too [9–11].

Occasionally, we have to deal with aphakic eyes. Several conditions can cause this entity, including congenital aphakia, trauma and intraoperative complications. While the first is rare we may see cases after congenital cataract surgery when no IOL was implanted in the first surgical procedure. The latter is sometimes associated with aniridia or large iris defects.

There exist numerous situations and different causes for IOL dislocation, IOL damage, IOL intolerance or aphakia. The design of an IOL and its optical characteristics are different in each case and so are the expectations of each individual patient. Hence, there is no standard treatment available that suits each individual patients' needs. Our aim as surgeons is to provide a tailored solution best suitable for each and every single patient.

Where the need arises, recentration of an IOL using scleral fixation combined with a flanging technique is a possible solution. Several options exist for refixation: we may flange the haptic directly or, use flanged sutures around a capsular tension ring (CTR), around IOL loops, haptic-eyelets or around holes in the IOL optic. By puncturing the IOL, we even may create holes within haptic or optic. In cases of misalignment of a toric add-on IOL we may rotate the implant in the sulcus and fixate it in the correct position with flanged sutures afterwards. We also may flange devices with sutures in order to support the capsular bag itself. In other cases where an IOL exchange may be advisable, the new IOL can be flanged to the sclera and finally we are confronted with aphakia and have to find the best solution.

In this chapter we aim to provide a systematic approach to facilitate the decision-making process when dealing with above mentioned conditions. We try to elucidate factors that help us in deciding whether refixation is an option or not, or whether IOL exchange is the better solution. We describe our specific approach for flanging techniques, utilizing specific instruments, also present different techniques for flanged scleral fixation in different situations of IOL dislocation and aphakia. Every surgeon has to find surgical solutions he or she is comfortable with, but there exist numerous surgical techniques and a plethora of instruments we can utilise. Even though it is absolutely impossible to mention all surgical techniques, implants and instruments available, this chapter should help each individual surgeon to adopt new ideas and help to find the best individual approach.

IOL Refixation or IOL Exchange

In some conditions refixation might be the best approach to treat cases with IOL luxation. In others, exchanging the whole IOL is the better option. What are the requirements for safe refixation?

Doubtlessly, it is mandatory that the implant has no evident damage. The optic should be transparent without any opacification [12, 13] and without severe damage after YAG capsulotomy [14]. Sometimes we may find cellular membranes on the IOL surface as signs of inferior uveal biocompatibility [15, 16].

These cells derive from monocytes and develop to foreign-body giant cells and fibroblast-like cells due to an ongoing intraocular inflammation. Hydrophilic IOLs may develop some calcification, especially after contact with air and gas tamponades [17–19].

We also should try to check the condition of the haptics. If we find bent or distorted haptics due to capsular shrinkage and biodegradation, IOL-exchange should be considered.

In every case we should gather as much information as possible about the implant. We can check, if an "IOL-pass" or a similar document is available or, if the IOL has such a typical design, that we can make a guess of the lens type. We also may ask at the institution where the patient was originally operated on or check the patients' notes if the patient was operated in our institution. With this information in hand we know, if the implant has a toric correction or if there are any other different optical features implemented into the IOL optic such as presbyopia correcting technology. Especially in the case of insufficient neuroadaptation or dysphotopsia after presbyopia correcting IOL implantation we may be forced to perform an IOL-exchange. In this case we have a certain risk of losing the option of safe IOL placement because of capsular problems [20–22].

With this information in hand we know the material of IOL optic and IOL haptic. In cases with 3-piece IOLs we need to know whether the haptic is made of PMMA or Polyvinylidenfluoride (PVDF). In such cases we might think about externalizing the haptics [23] and flanging them using a modified Yamane technique [1].

In single-piece IOLs with closed loops we might use the eyelet or the hole of the closed loop for a double flanged suture fixation. A modified Canabrava technique might be a valuable option in such cases [24]. Even in some cases with open loop IOLs we may be able to re-fixate the capsule/IOL compartment with double flanged sutures or in the case of an eyelet using one flange right at the eyelet and the other end at the sclera.

In certain specific situations we may even create holes to the IOL and fixate it with sutures by flanging one suture end at the site of the artificial IOL hole and the other suture end to the sclera as Assia described previously [25]. Even a fibrotic capsular rim may be used as scuffold for an IOL refixation.

In cases of misalignment of a toric add-on IOL we may fixate the sulcus implant with flanged sutures aiming at a corrected alignment of the IOL axis.

If we find a capsular tension ring (CTR) within the capsule/IOL compartment we may be able to use the ring for refixation using flanged polypropylene sutures for scleral fixation again.

Apart from an undamaged IOL as a prerequisite for refixation it is also advisable to exchange the IOL together with the capsular bag in cases of severe intracapsular proliferation and calcification (Soemmering ring) [26, 27]. Particularly in this situation the haptics may be damaged by myofibroblastic metaplasia of lens epithelial cells, causing distortion of haptics and leading to a loss of the shape memory effect [28, 29].

Another issue might arise from proliferative lens-material floating from the capsular bag into the vitreous cavity after puncture of the capsule during the surgical maneuvers, causing floaters, uveitis or glaucoma. We may refixate an IOL within a capsular bag filled with lens-material too, but preferably, we are confronted with a dead bag syndrome [30], with an almost empty, clear capsular bag and an IOL without any damage for our refixation strategy.

Because of all the factors mentioned above, it is mandatory to describe each single situation in detail in order to discuss the best approach for refixation or for exchange of the IOL.

IOL Dislocation Without Capsular Support

This rare situation may occur as an intraoperative complication when the IOL is luxated posteriorly into the vitreous cavity and the capsule does not give sufficient support for IOL repositioning into the bag or in the sulcus. If the implant used during the primary surgery was a 3-piece IOL then refixation of the IOL seems to be the most atraumatic solution.

After thorough pars plana vitrectomy with 3 scleral ports the retina is inspected for retinal tears under indentation. In case of retinal breaks retinopexy is performed using endolaser. One haptic is grasped carefully with a vitreoretinal-forceps and lifted. There are two options to proceed. One option is to grasp the haptic end in the vitreous cavity directly (Fig. 1), to externalize one haptic 2 mm from the limbus through a 2 mm long tunnel and to flange it (Fig. 2). The same maneuver is performed with the second haptic on the contralateral side thereafter (Fig. 3). Grasping the IOL within the vitreous cavity provides more space for the maneuvers and any contact of the IOL with tissue in the anterior chamber is avoided. The externalization can be achieved with a 27G or 30G thin walled needle or with the Amon forceps-needle (FN) [1, 31]. Both haptics flanged, we position the IOL by pushing the haptic ends towards the sclera applying some pressure in order to use the flanges as some kind of a plug inside the very end of the scleral tunnel and to bury the flanges below the conjunctiva and Tenons layer.

The second option is to bring the IOL into the anterior chamber first and to position it there for further manipulation (Fig. 4). From there externalization and flanging starts in the anterior chamber, similar to the classical Yamane technique (Fig. 5).

In cases with closed loops after pp VE the IOL may be lifted and positioned into the anterior chamber. As positioning the sutures through the haptics within the vitreous cavity seems to be more difficult, this maneuver should be undertaken within the anterior chamber. It might be advisable to use some viscoelatic for endothelial protection during this procedure. By titrating the infusion pressure, care has to be taken, similar to a malignant glaucoma reaction, that a posterior blockage resulting in a collapse of the anterior chamber is avoided. A flanging

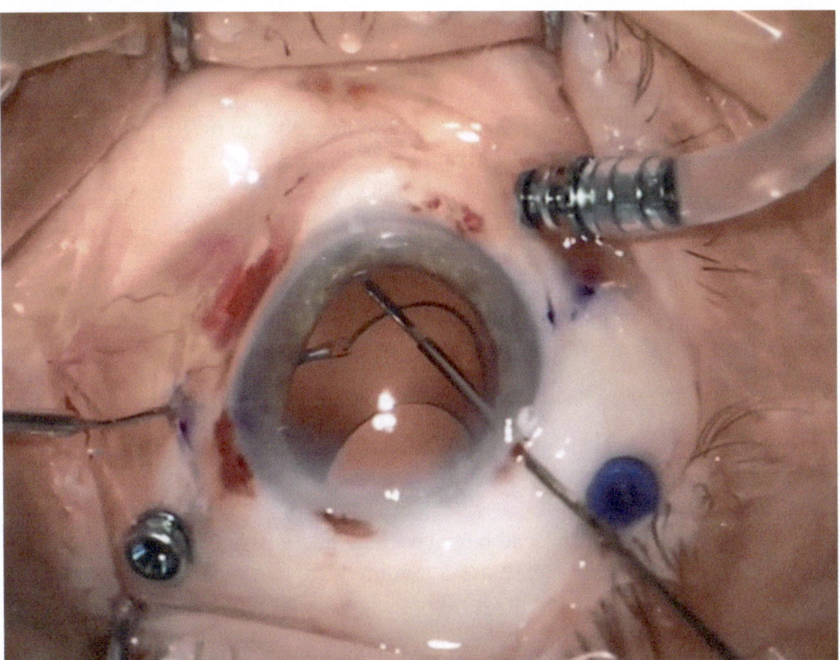

Fig. 1 Grasping of the first haptic-end with the FN in the vitreous cavity

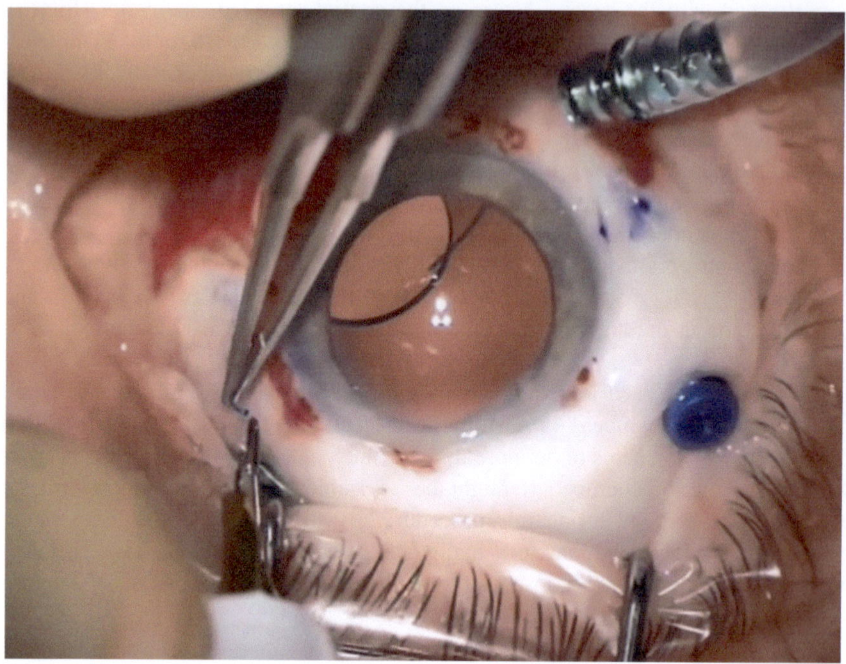

Fig. 2 Flanging of the first haptic-end (PMMA)

technique with 6-0 polypropylene sutures (alternatively 5-0 or 7-0 sutures may be used) may be applied for scleral refixation.

With all these techniques mentioned above we just need scleral ports and a limbal side port. As we avoid IOL-exchange with this technique, we do not need any main incision for IOL implantation.

In cases with IOLs not suitable for refixation it is advisable to explant the luxated IOL. As soon as the IOL is explanted, after vitrectomy we may implant the new IOL best suited for our preferred flanging technique.

3-Piece IOL in an Almost Empty Capsular Bag (Dead Bag Syndrome): Refixation by Flanging the Two Haptics

If we face a situation with a dead bag syndrome and a 3-piece IOL with PMMA- or polypropylene haptics we may use a modified Yamane technique for refixation of the IOL/capsule compartment. As this technique is more demanding a scleral port for infusion is recommended. With the scleral port a sufficient vitrectomy behind the IOL can be performed and, if needed the whole capsular bag and its content can be removed after refixation.

Depending on the position of the haptic ends of the dislocated IOL, the site for preparation for the scleral tunnel is determined in order to minimize intraocular

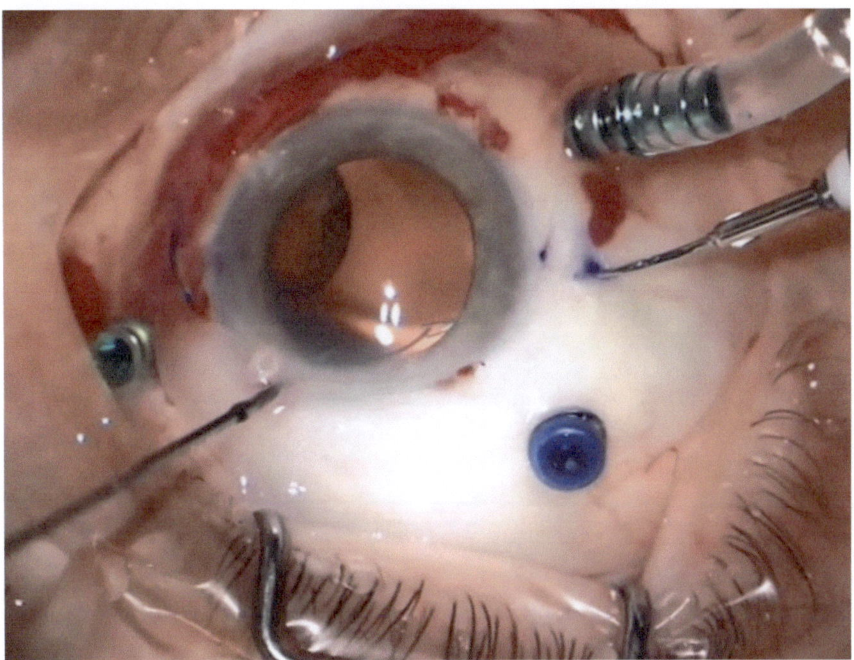

Fig. 3 Grasping of the second haptic-end before externalisation

IOL rotation. While stabilising the eye with a forceps, 2 mm from the limbus the FN creates the first scleral tunnel about 2 mm in length. With a bimanuel maneuver the capsular equator or an accessible part of the IOL is grasped by forceps and the FN punctures the capsular equator at the site of one haptic end (Fig. 6). As soon as the capsule equator is opened the FN may prepare the haptic end, grasp it and can externalize the first haptic. The haptic end is then flanged. Now the second tunnel is prepared with the FN in the same manner 180 degrees to the first tunnel. Using the second forceps to hold the capsular bag and IOL in a stable position the capsular equator can be punctured more easily (Fig. 7). The second haptic end is grasped finally, externalized and flanged. The haptic ends are pressed against the external part of the scleral tunnel, so that they are covered by the conjunctiva and Tenons layer sufficiently.

After flanged refixation of the IOL, the capsular bag and the lens-material inside the capsular bag may be removed with a vitreous cutter, followed by thorough vitrectomy via the scleral port (Fig. 8).

As this technique seems to be quite challenging, especially in conditions with a capsular bag filled with a huge amount of lens-material, alternatively an IOL exchange may be considered in such cases.

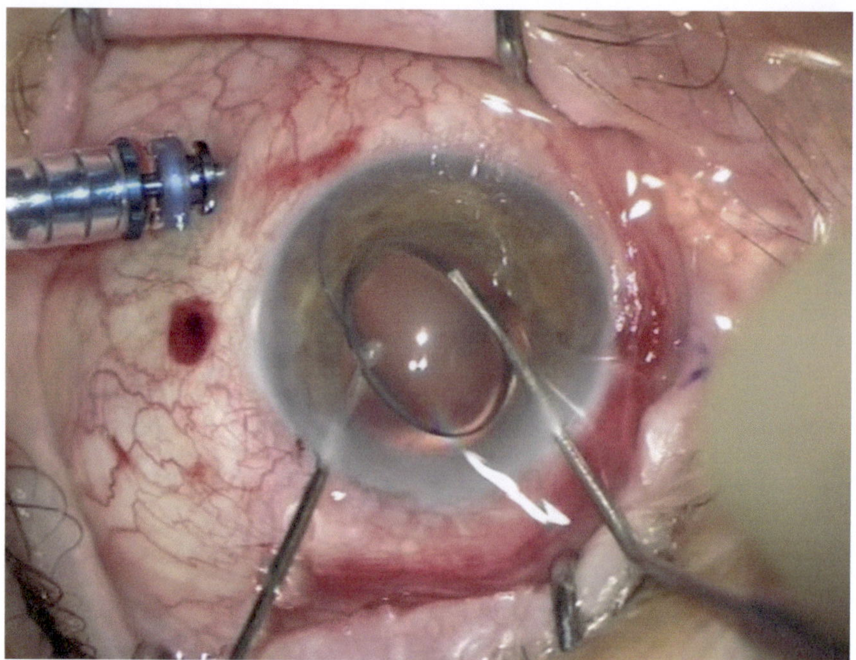

Fig. 4 Rotation and positioning of the IOL in the anterior chamber

IOL/Capsule Compartment Plus CTR in an Almost Empty Capsular Bag (Dead Bag Syndrome): Refixation with Double Flanged Sutures

If the IOL/capsule compartment contains a CTR we are in a favourable situation, as we may flange sutures around the CTR. This is the reason why in all my pseudoexfoliation (PEX) cataract cases I primarily implant a CTR, so that in case of a late onset dislocation after years I can use the described technique for refixation. If there is no severe proliferative material within the capsular bag, described as dead bag syndrome, refixation seems the best solution in these cases, no matter if the posterior capsule has been opened previously with YAG-capsulotomy or not.

In cases of vitreous presence in the anterior chamber an anterior vitrectomy should be performed initially. This is easily done bimanually via two 1 mm limbal incisions. In cases with a CTR an infusion via anterior chamber maintainer or scleral port is not mandatory, but might facilitate the surgical maneuvers. In this case we need to control the infusion pressure closely, as we might induce a collapse of the anterior chamber by using an infusion. This situation can be caused by a capsular block syndrome. In this case clearance of the anterior vitreous is mandatory in order to overcome the posterior block syndrome. Afterwards a perpendicular scleral perforation with the FN is performed 2.5 mm away from the limbus. Some surgeons prepare a limbus parallel tunnel for the suture fixation.

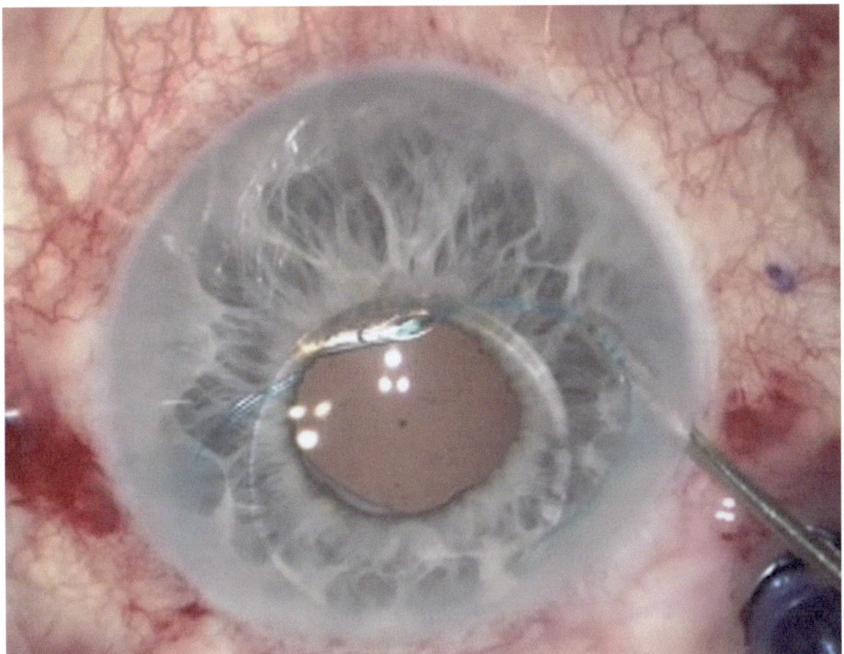

Fig. 5 Grasping of the haptic-end (PMMA) in the anterior chamber

This might be especially useful in cases with a very thin sclera. One disadvantage of this method is that we only can estimate the length of the tunnel and do not know the exact exit of the needle inside the eye. With the FN we then perforate the posterior sheet of the capsule behind the CTR and perforate the anterior sheet of the capsule (Fig. 9). With the second hand we bring a 6-0 polypropylene suture into the anterior chamber and externalize the suture with the FN (Fig. 10). I prefer the 6-0 version for flanging, as smaller dimensions may slide through the scleral tunnel and might have a higher incidence of biodegradation. The "rail road" or "hand shake" technique may be applied alternatively, guiding the suture out of the eye with a bent needle [32].

Then the same maneuver is performed anterior to the CTR (Fig. 11). 1.5–2.0 mm from the limbus, on the same axis as the first scleral tunnel, a perpendicular scleral perforation is created and the second end of the suture is grasped and externalized with the FN again. Now one end of the suture is flanged and positioned under the conjunctiva. By pulling the second end the IOL/capsule compartment is centered and it is intended to create some tension to the suture. Then the suture is grasped as close to the sclera as possible and is cut about 1.5 mm from the forceps with scissors. The suture is trimmed thereafter in the way that the short free second end is flanged towards the holding forceps. As it is intended that the sutures are under some, moderate tension, after giving the suture free the second suture end will slide behind the conjunctiva and Tenons layer and will stop at the

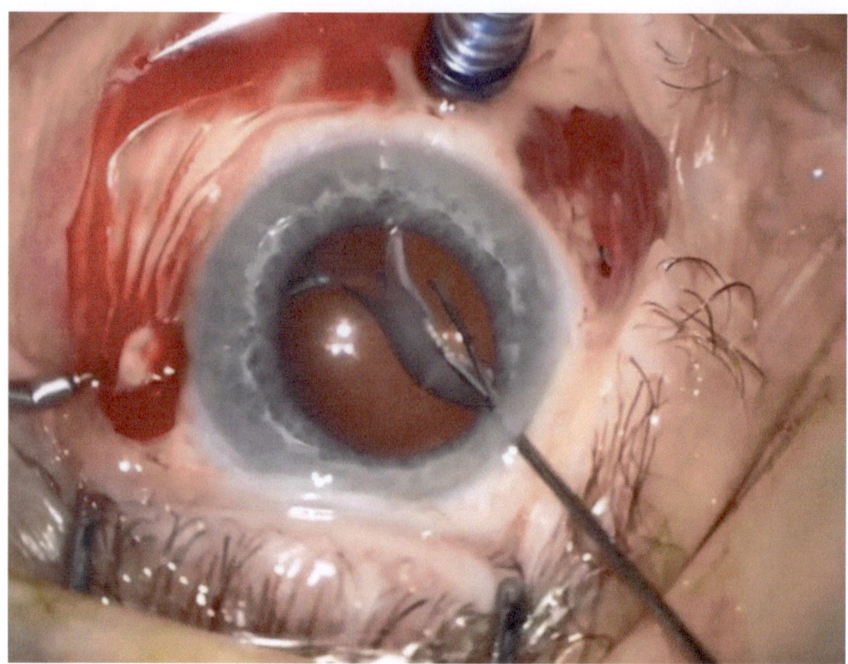

Fig. 6 Stabilisation of the IOL and puncture of the capsule equator close to the haptic-end (PMMA)

entry of the scleral tunnel. Finally conjunctiva and Tenons layer are actively elevated above the flanges. In some cases a single double flanged suture is enough for appropriate centration and fixation (Fig. 12), as parts of the persistent zonular complex and of the capsular bag hold the IOL in position too.

If adequate centration and fixation cannot be achieved by a single suture, this procedure should be performed on the contralateral side or on any other side of the CTR again (Fig. 13). Applying a 3-point fixation with double flanged sutures we may preclude any tilt of the CTR/IOL compartment.

By forced movements of the eye with forceps, we can test if the IOL is positioned safely and is not wobbling anymore. In all these cases the capsular bag should not be removed, as together with the suture the capsular bag holds the CTR and the IOL in place.

IOL with Closed Haptic-Loops in an Almost Empty Capsular Bag (Dead Bag Syndrome): Refixation with Double Flanged Sutures

In cases with an almost empty capsule, no CTR but closed haptic-loops or haptic-eyelets we may use a similar technique of double flanged suture fixation. We can use the openings of the closed loops or eyelets for flanged suture refixation. We

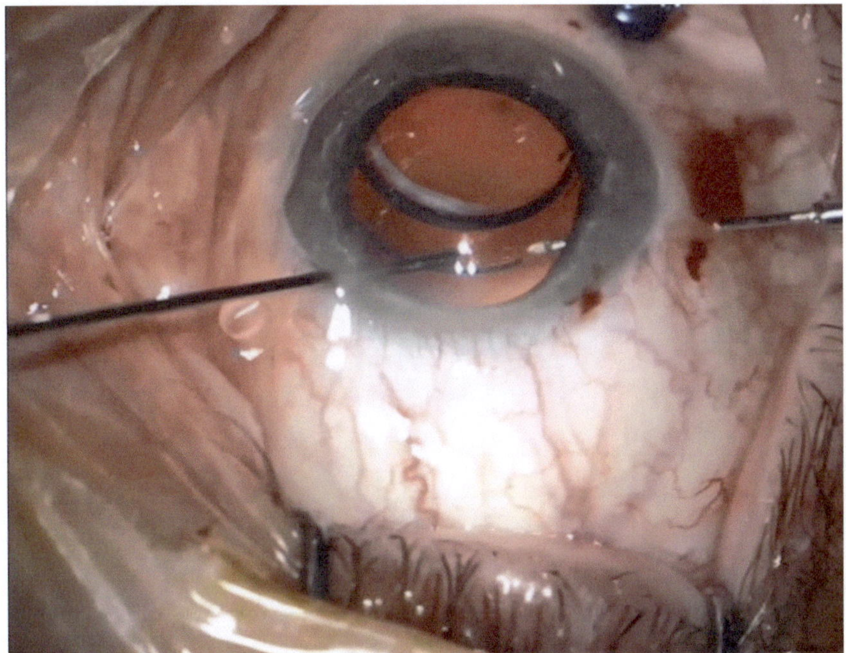

Fig. 7 Stabilisation of the IOL and puncture of the capsule with the FN close to the second haptic-end

can use the FN again or a plain needle to puncture the sclera and the capsule and to externalize the polypropylene suture. 2.5 mm from the limbus a scleral tunnel is prepared and the FN perforates the posterior capsule behind the IOL, is advanced through the haptic-loop or eyelet and perforates the anterior capsule Fig. 14. With the second forceps the 6-0 polypropylene suture is introduced into the anterior chamber and grasped and externalised with the FN. After perpendicular or limbus parallel scleral tunnel preparation the second suture-end is externalized from the anterior chamber 1.5–2.0 mm from the limbus above the IOL haptic Fig. 15.

This procedure may be applied on the contralateral side again. Centration of the IOL is controlled and changed by the tension of the sutures at the final stage. While holding and lifting the sutures close to the sclera, all the suture ends are flanged. If we need to overcome an IOL tilt, we may apply a 3 point double flanged suture fixation. As there is some faint tension applied to the sutures during the flanging maneuver and by the IOL itself, conjunctival erosion does not occur with this technique. As the flanges slide into the external opening of the scleral tunnel, they may work like a plug. The tunnels remain watertight even though the tunnels are relatively short, in case of a perpendicular scleral preparation.

The position of the double flanged sutures is given by the position of the haptic loops. As we should avoid rotating the IOL too much within the eye, we should try to thread the sutures at the position of the haptic-loops. If the IOL was toric,

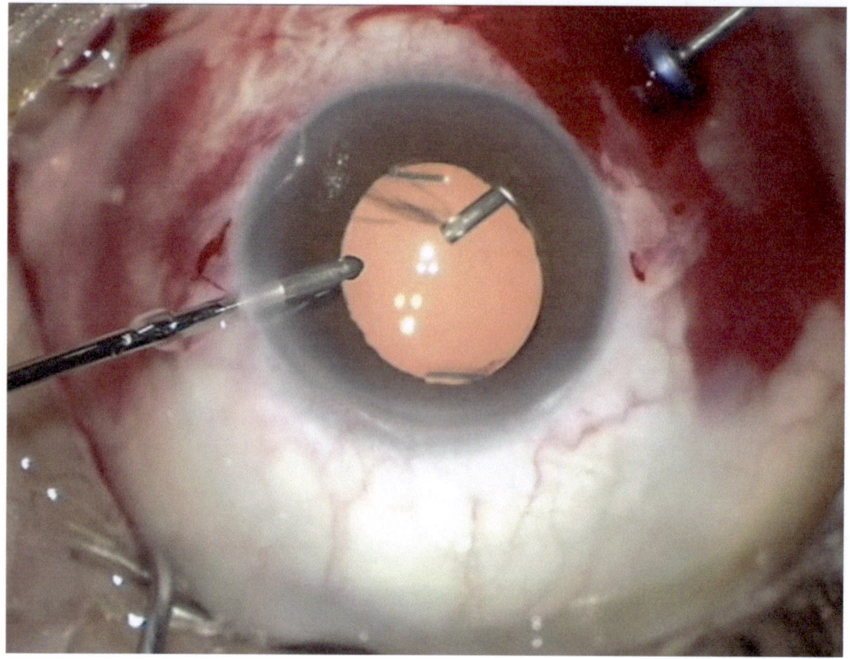

Fig. 8 Thorough vitrectomy and capsulectomy via the scleral port

the alignment of the IOL has to be taken into consideration. Centration of the IOL is influenced by the tension of the sutures applied towards the IOL and can be determined by the surgeon. By adding a third suture a 3-point fixation can influence the IOL tilt and may minimise it.

Fixation of Ocular Tissue or of Intraocular Devices with Flanging Techniques

Some situations exist where it might be advisable to refixate the capsular bag in order to implant the IOL into the capsular bag thereafter. Especially in cases with extensive intraoperative zonular dehiscence or with diffuse weakness of the zonular apparatus we may use CTRs with eyelets [24, 33] or alternatiely an anchor [34] for capsule stabilization. With this technique we may avoid vitreous loss and hopefully can avoid vitrectomy. All these devices can be fixated to the sclera utilizing flanged polypropylene sutures. In these cases it is advisable to thread the suture through the eyelet before implantation. One end of the suture is flanged with cautery and it is tested that the flange is not sliding through the eyelet. Now the device is implanted and brought into position. Then the second end of the suture is externalized with the FN or with a needle utilizing the "rail road" or "hand shake" technique [32]. By pulling the external end of the suture the device is positioned and the capsular bag

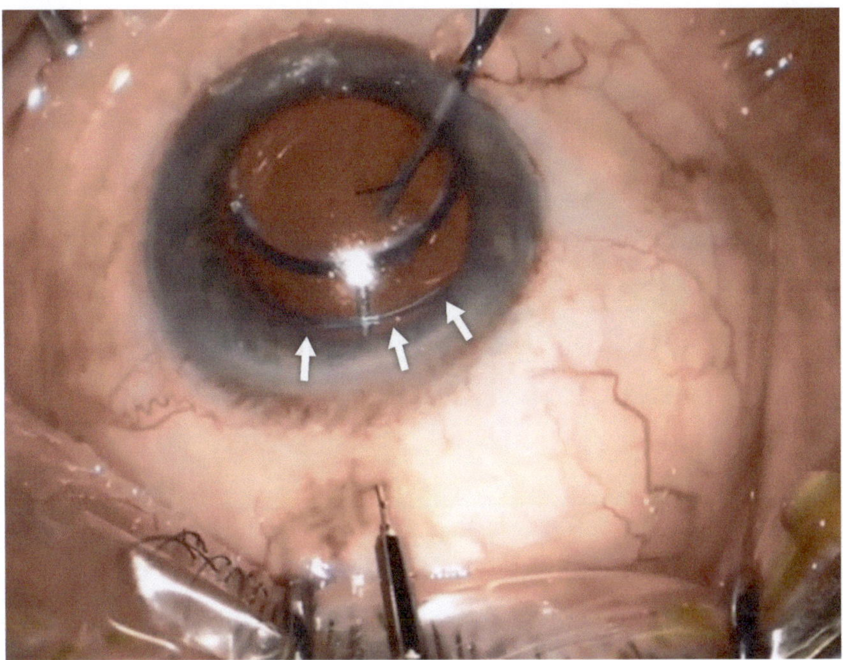

Fig. 9 FN behind the CTR, puncturing posterior and anterior capsule; 6-0 polypropylene suture before externalisation

secured. Now we grasp the suture close to the sclera, cut the suture about 1.5 mm from the forceps and create a flange. Usually when we open the forceps, as there was some tension applied to the suture, the flange glides through the conjunctiva and stops at the sclera. With this technique we achieve a watertight, safe flange position. The flange functions as plug and is covered by conjunctiva. In Chap. 5 similar techniques are described in detail. The capsular bag secured and fixated to the sclera serves in its original function again and will hold the IOL in position.

In the case of a posterior capsule rupture it is widely accepted to implant a 3-piece IOL into the sulcus with the option to position the optic behind the existing capsulorhexis. Even in cases with anterior radial tears of the capsule transequatorially extending to the posterior capsule or in cases with lokalised zonular dehiscence we can position the IOL in the sulcus without any suture fixation. But if the zonular defect is too large for safe sulcus placement of the IOL, we have to secure the IOL with sutures. We may remove the remnants of the capsule and proceed with our flanging technique as in any aphakic case or we may asymmetrically flange one part of the IOL and use the capsular remnants for stabilisation of the second haptic. Flanging one haptic end of a 3-piece IOL to the sclera and positioning the second haptic on top of the capsular remnant in the sulcus would result in a significant decentration of the IOL. In this situation there exists an interesting technique utilizing a 6-0 polypropylene suture in combination

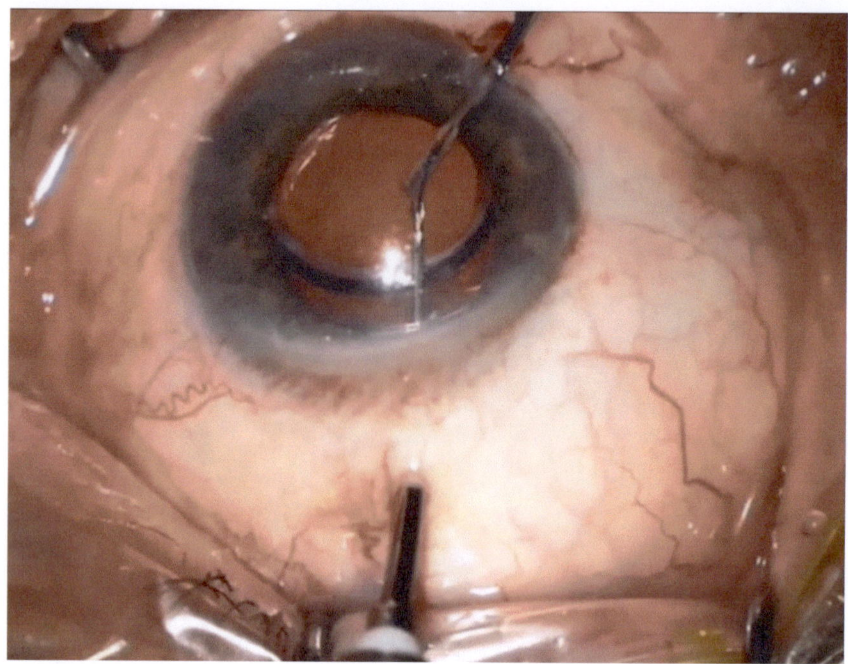

Fig. 10 Grasping the first suture-end with the FN right before externalisation

with a flanged haptic of a 3-piece IOL. First a flange is created to the first end of the suture. Immediately after the flanging, the material still hot and workable, the flange is pressed into a flat, paddleshaped form with forceps. Then a hole is made through the flattened flange and one haptic end is threaded through the created eyelet. Now the end of this haptic is flanged, so that the suture cannot slide out from the haptic. After implantation of the IOL with injector or with forceps the second suture end is externalized 2.0 mm from the limbus at the contralateral side of the capsular remnants. Having positioned the second haptic behind the iris on top of the capsule the IOL is centered by pulling the suture outside the eye. As soon as the IOL is in position the suture is trimmed about 1.5 mm from the sclera, flanged and positioned behind the iris. With this technique we only need a single suture flange for scleral fixation, as the haptic flange only works as a barrier precluding slippage of the haptic through the eyelet of the suture.

Even in the rare circumstances of aniridia or large iris defects an artificial iris may be flanged to the sclera with polypropylene sutures or by flanged haptics of a 3-piece IOL [35, 36], additional Citation: Novel surgical techniquenof a sutureless artificial iris and intraocular lens scleral fixation using Yamane technique; D. Muth, S. Priglinger, M Shajari et al. Am. J. Ophthalmol Case reports 26 (2022) 101502. Double flanged sutures may also be used for the fixation of ocular tissue (iris) to the sclera, e.g. in the case of an iridodialysis (Fig. 16).

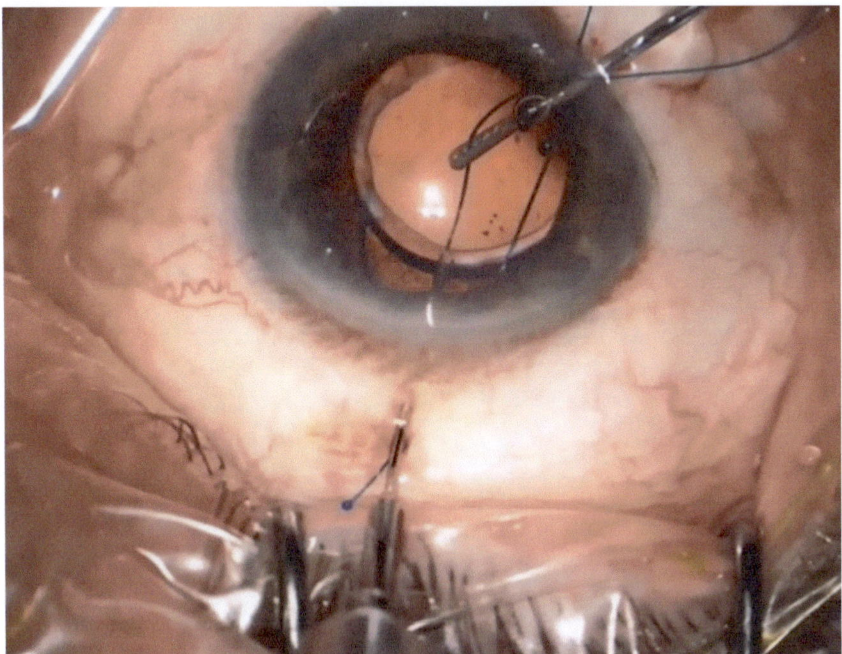

Fig. 11 Externalisation of the second suture-end above the CTR; first suture-end is flanged already

On Axis Fixation of Add-On IOLs After Misalignment

As toric or multifocal/toric add-on IOLs are not held in position by capsular structures because of their position in the ciliary sulcus, misalignment caused by IOL rotation may occur at any time after surgery. The incidence of add-on IOL rotation of more than 10 degrees is about 10% [37, 38].

In case of rotation of the IOL single re-positioning may again be followed by a misalignment at a later stage. A flanging technique can be applied in such a case, too. In this situation the correct axis is marked with any preferred technique first. For fixation of the add-on IOL 9-0 or 8-0 polypropylene sutures armed with a spatula needle are strong enough to hold the lens in place as the forces to counteract the tendency of rotation are very low. Under OVD and with two side ports the add-on IOL is rotated, aligned to the correct axis and the non-armed end of the suture is flanged. The add-on IOL is held with forceps and a 30G needle is preparing a perpendicular scleral tunnel at the site of the marked axis behind the iris. The optic periphery or the haptic-end is then perforated with the spatula needle of the suture at the site of the toric IOL mark or at the haptic-end and pushed into the opening of the 30G needle and externalized (Fig. 17).

By pulling the suture through the add-on IOL the trailing flange is positioned at the optic periphery or at the haptic-end of the toric add-on IOL. With some

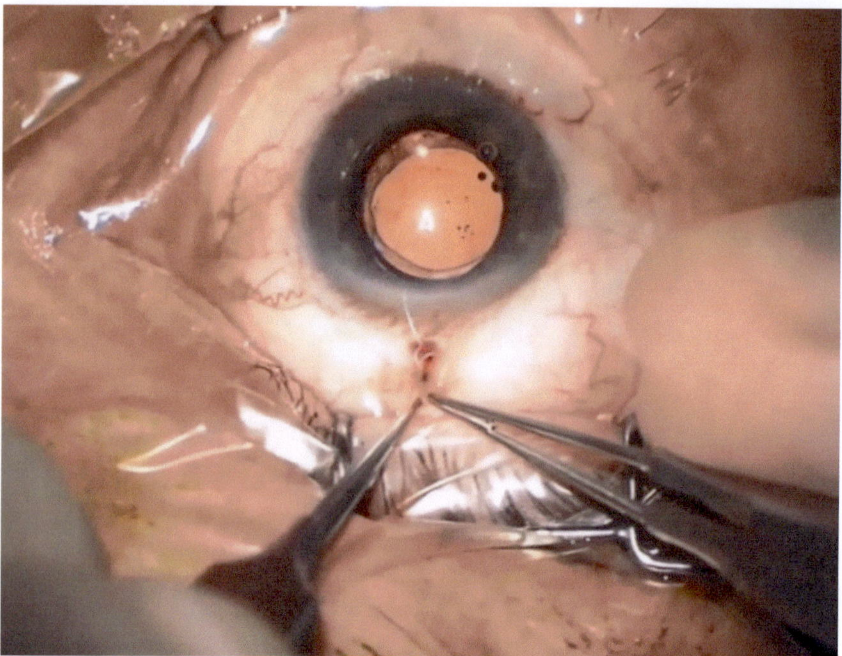

Fig. 12 Well centered and stable position of the IOL after a single double flanged suture fixation

tension, taking care not to decenter the IOL the suture is held close to the sclera and cut about 1.5 mm from the forceps. The external suture may then be flanged with cautery and positioned under the conjunctiva. Alternatively, a zig-zag fixation could be performed for scleral IOL fixation without the need to create a knot [39]. In order to keep the IOL in position a single fixation suture seems to be sufficient enough.

IOL-Exchange

As mentioned above all dislocated IOLs with obvious damage to the implant are recommended to be exchanged. The same applies for all cases with severe alteration of the capsular bag such as a Soemmering ring formation. In this case we find masses of proliferative material partly calcified, located in the periphery of the capsular bag. This often coincides with torn and bent haptics, having lost their memory over the time. The biodegradation is often reinforced by the myofibroblastic metaplasia of lens epithelial cells. In all these cases explantation of the IOL/capsule compartment is the best approach. After explantation and thorough vitrectomy the IOL of choice may be implanted and flanged with our favored technique.

Sometimes there is no IOL dislocation forcing us to exchange the IOL. Damage or opacification of the IOL optic, refractory membranes on the IOL surface or

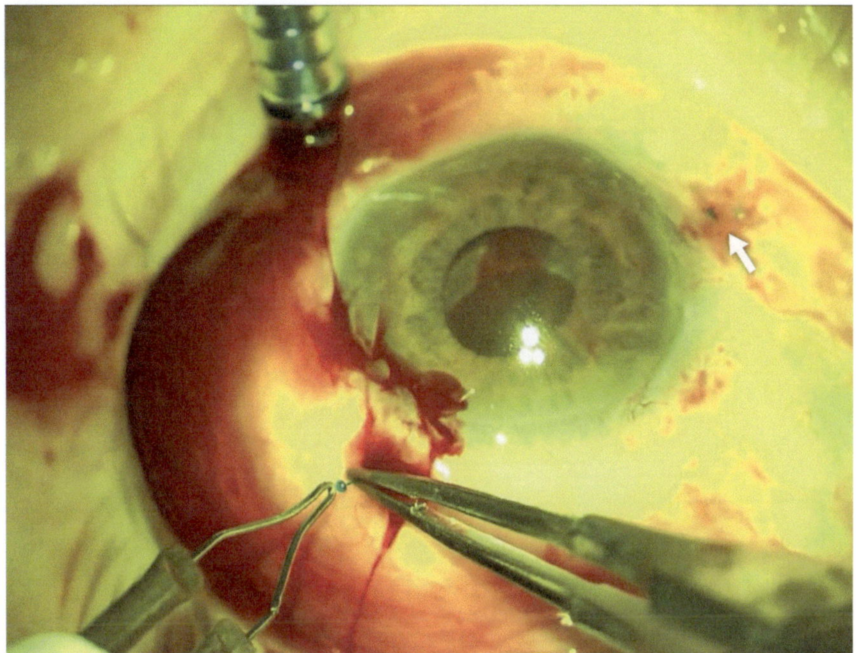

Fig. 13 Fixation of the CTR/IOL compartment with two double flanged polypropylene sutures (anticoagulant therapy)

massive pseudophakodonesis make IOL explantation necessary [12, 13]. Other causes for explantation are a biometrical surprise, severe dysphotopsia or lack of neuroadaptation, especially in cases after multifocal IOL implantation [40–44]. Usually we are able to preserve the capsular bag for proper in the bag placement of an IOL. However during explantation we might realize that the capsular bag or the zonular apparatus are compromised and safe IOL placement becomes impossible. In these rare cases an IOL exchange combined with a flanging technique can be used.

In the case of IOL exchange a scleral infusion is very helpful as it facilitates vitrectomy. Furthermore, a fluid current from posterior to anterior lifts the implant anteriorly. After positioning the scleral infusion two side ports and a 2.4 to 2.8 mm incision, dependent on the incision size needed for the IOL to be implanted, are prepared. Numerous techniques exist for IOL explantation, depending on IOL material, IOL design and personal preference.

Our routine technique is to hold the IOL/capsule compartment with forceps and to cut the IOL in two pieces (Fig. 18). Afterwards, the capsular bag and its content are explanted in total. Often the material inside the capsular bag slides out of the capsular bag and stays within the eye. As the calcified parts cannot be removed with the vitreous cutter easily and the soft material cannot be grasped by forceps, most of the material may passively be discharged via the main incision (Fig. 19).

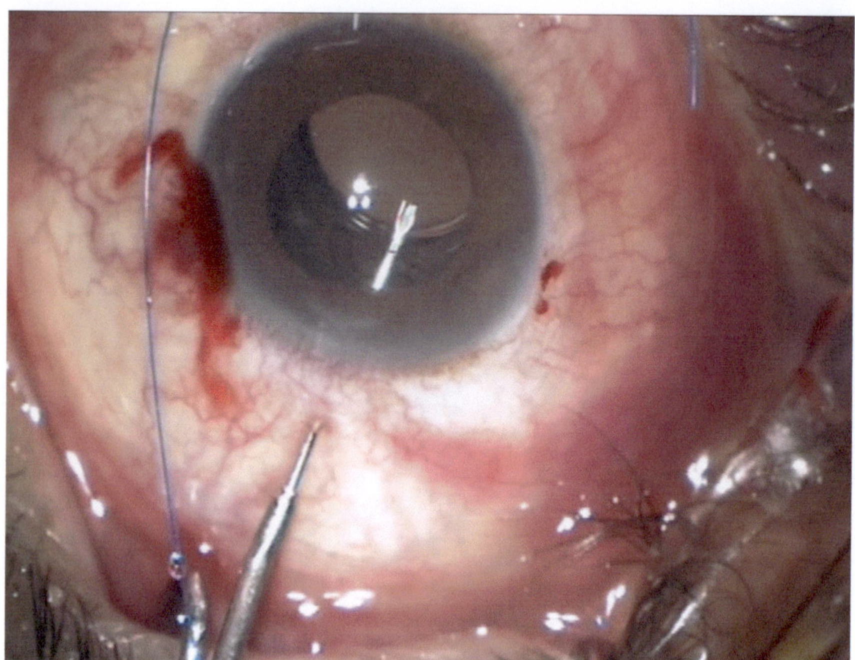

Fig. 14 After puncture of the posterior capsule the FN is threaded through the closed loop of the IOL

Utilizing the current of the infusion fluid due to the pressure gradient, by lifting the main incision, most of the material will float out from the eye. Usually the remaining part can be either removed by forceps or by a cutter. If it is not possible to remove the lensmaterial with a cutter, it sometimes is advisable to aspirate the lensmaterial with the cutter and to guide the material out through the main incision. Alternatively an IOL injector may be used to aspirate the lensmaterial. In case of luxation of lens material into the vitreous cavity a 3-port pars plana vitrectomy has to be performed.

In all cases thorough anterior vitrectomy is mandatory to avoid vitreoretinal complications and to preclude vitreoretinal traction during IOL fixation.

After thorough anterior vitrectomy the IOL of choice is implanted through the main incision thereafter. Chapters 3, 4 and 5 describe the flanging techniques applicable in detail. In Chap. 7 IOLs suitable for flanging techniques are listed. Basically, we have the option of flanging haptics of 3-piece IOLs made of PMMA or preferably PVDF. In this case we may externalize the haptics with a thin-walled needle or with the FN.

Another option is the externalization and flanging of polypropylene sutures. Depending on the technique we choose, we have to decide which type of IOL we use. The type of IOL itself determines the technique of implantation and the wound-size.

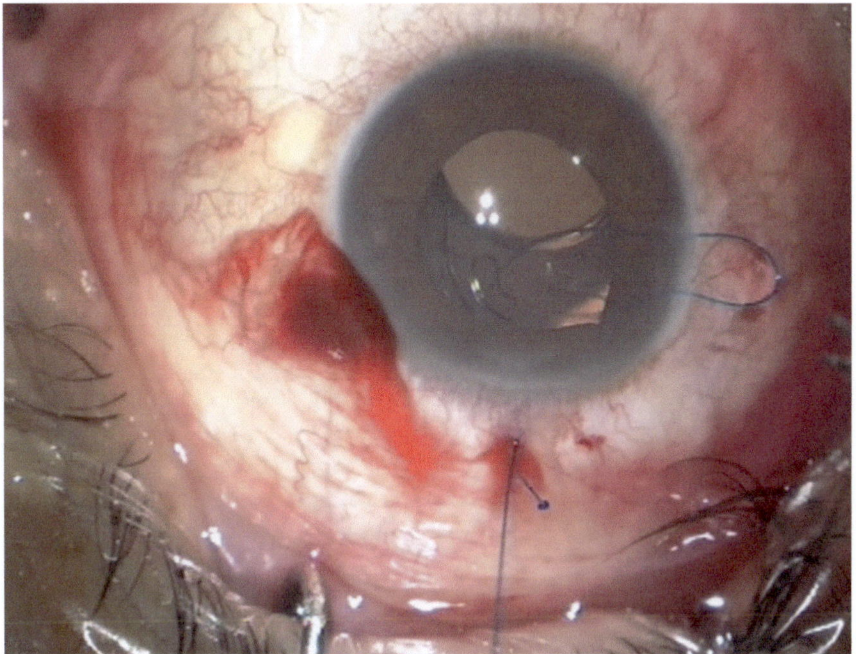

Fig. 15 The polypropylene suture is tightened before flanging of the second suture-end

Correction of Aphakia

As described in the previous chapter there are many solutions to rehabilitate patients with aphakia independent of the underlying cause. In almost all cases implantation of an IOL will represent the best option. When we want to apply a technique with implantation of a posterior IOL combined with flanging haptics or sutures a wide pupil for better visualization during surgery is one key to success. In cases of aphakia an active infusion is helpful to keep the eye pressure stable. Depending on the individual preference we may use an anterior chamber maintainer or a scleral port for the intraocular infusion. Personally, I prefer a scleral infusion. With this approach the anterior chamber is less crowded and vitrectomy can be performed more sufficiently.

If we face a situation with sufficient capsular support for safe IOL placement to the sulcus, scleral flanging may not be needed. However, in doubtful cases with an unknown capsular condition we should apply a flanging technique. It is recommended to perform an anterior vitrectomy in all cases. Capsular remnants should be removed as well. For implantation of our selected IOL we need a main incision and should prepare two side-ports additionally.

The next steps depend on the flanging technique used. We have the option to use the Yamane technique and flange the two haptics or to use the Canabrava technique

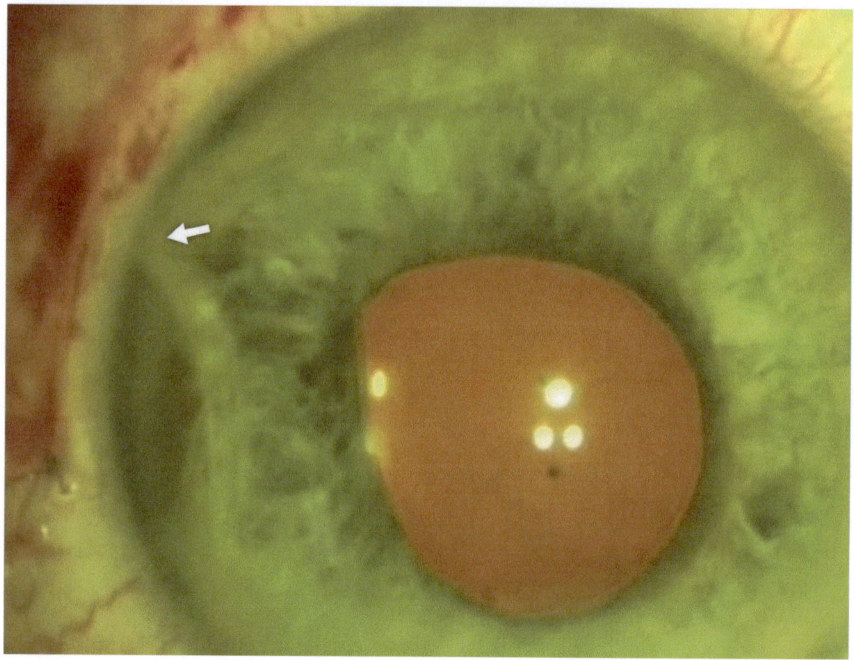

Fig. 16 Scleral irisfixation with a double flanged polypropylene suture after traumatic iridodialysis

and flange the ends of a polypropylene suture. Both techniques are described in Chaps. 3 and 4 in detail.

There exist a lot of variations for the Yamane technique, from the classical technique utilising two thin-walled 30 G needles with simultaenous externalisation to sequential externalisation with needles. Some surgeons externalize the trailing haptic first and position the leading haptic contralateral to the main incision therefor. Mainly a superior incision is used, but a temporal incision can be used either.

When we apply the Yamane technique my approach is as follows: we mark the entry site of the scleral tunnels 2 mm from the limbus away with a caliper at the axis we want to fixate the IOL (horizontal, vertical or on steep axis in case of toric IOL). A scleral port is positioned, the infusion is set at moderate height and two side ports and the 2.4 mm limbal main incision are prepared. A 3-piece IOL with PVDF haptics is implanted and the leading haptic is positioned in the anterior chamber. The trailing haptic is kept outside the incision first. Now the scleral tunnel is prepared with the FN, holding the eye close to the incision at the limbus with surgical forceps. Before tunnel preparation the conjunctiva is moved away from the entry site, so that after the flanging procedure unharmed conjunctiva covers the flange. The tunnel should be approximately 2 mm long. Then the FN is advanced and turned so that it becomes visible in the pupillary area. A bent holding forceps is introduced into the anterior chamber at one side port and the

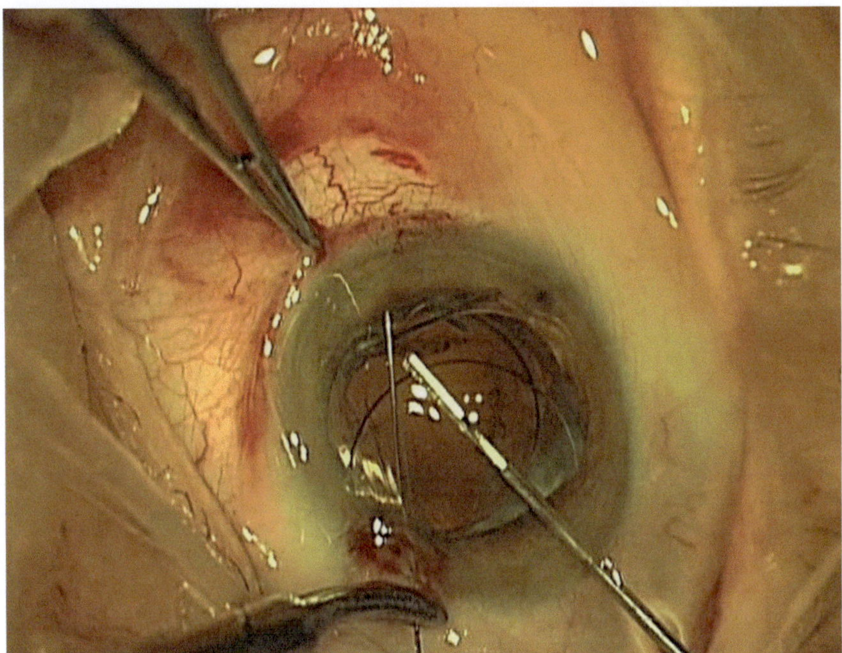

Fig. 17 Perforation of the haptic-end of a toric add-on IOL with the spatula needle of a 9-0 polypropylene suture

leading haptic is grasped about 3 mm from its end. The haptic end is now grasped by the FN (Fig. 20). Even though 100% alignment of haptic and needle is not mandatory for grasping, it is advisable to optimize the working angle of haptic and FN. The ideal position to grasp the haptic is such that its end is positioned at the very beginning of the needle, behind the two branches of the forceps. After grasping the haptic is then slowly externalized. The end of the haptic is dried with a sponge and flanged with a low temperature dry cautery. It is important not to touch the haptic with the cautery as it will stick to it and complicate further maneuvers. The optic is then gently pushed behind the iris with a spatula. On the contralateral side the second scleral tunnel is prepared with the FN in the same manner. The trailing haptic is grasped with the forceps, introduced and grasped by the FN. Even if haptic-end and FN are not at an ideal angle, the end may be grasped sufficiently enough to continue (Fig. 21). After externalization the flange is prepared in the same way as mentioned above. The haptic ends are brought into position and gently pressed against the scleral tunnel. Ideally, the flanges are covered by unharmed conjunctiva and Tenons layer and embedded in the external part of the scleral wound. Finally, the position of the IOL is inspected. In case of decentration the haptics can be shortened in order to optimize the IOL position.

Similar to other techniques there exist many modifications of the Canabrava technique. The described variation is our preferred technique, but as long as the

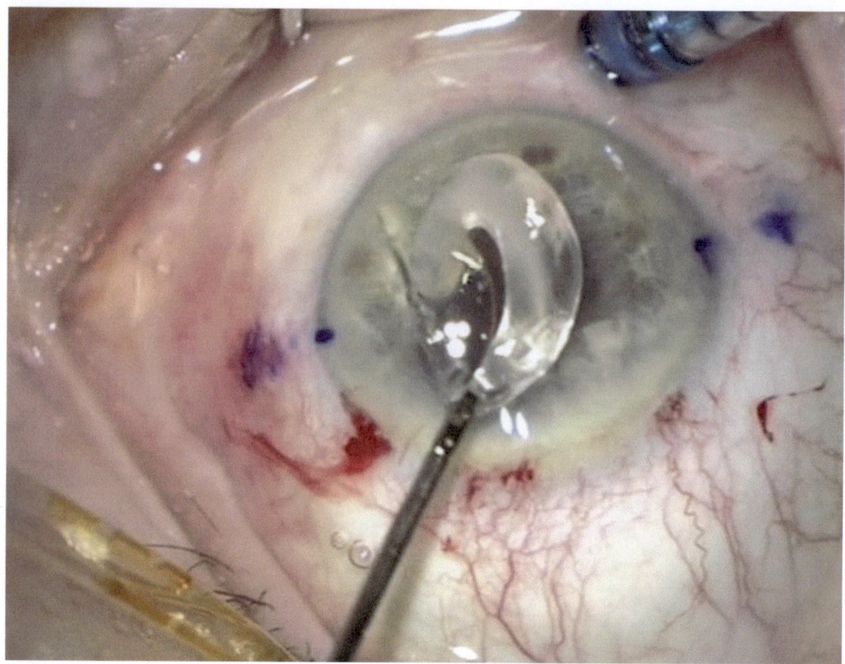

Fig. 18 Explantation of the first part of the cut IOL and of parts of the capsule with its capsular remnants

principles of this technique are preserved, they can be modified in different ways at will.

For the Canabrava technique [24] the entry sites for the FN are marked 2 mm from the limbus with a circle at our preferred axis of fixation. The two scleral incisions needed for the double flanged technique of one side are marked at a distance of 5 mm. A scleral port or an anterior chamber maintainer is positioned, the infusion is set at 40 cm and two side ports and a 3.2 mm limbal incision are prepared. Now the leading two closed loop haptics are threaded with the first 6-0 polypropylene suture symmetrically (Fig. 22). Personally, I prefer to implant the folded IOL with forceps but there exist different techniques including the use of an injector. The IOL is brought into the anterior chamber, both suture ends are cut for further comfortable manipulation and grasped by forceps. After moving the conjunctiva to the side, the FN is introduced through the first perpendicular scleral tunnel, the first end of the suture is grasped and externalized (Fig. 23). A limbus parallel scleral tunnel may be prepared alternatively to a perpendicular scleral tunnel preparation. 6-0 polypropylene sutures are quite rigid. Hence, it is advisable to grasp them with the FN similar to haptics at their very end as grasping the suture in between sometimes will not allow the suture to fold and slide into the hollow needle. Instead, they might slide out the FN entirely. The same procedure is performed with the second end now.

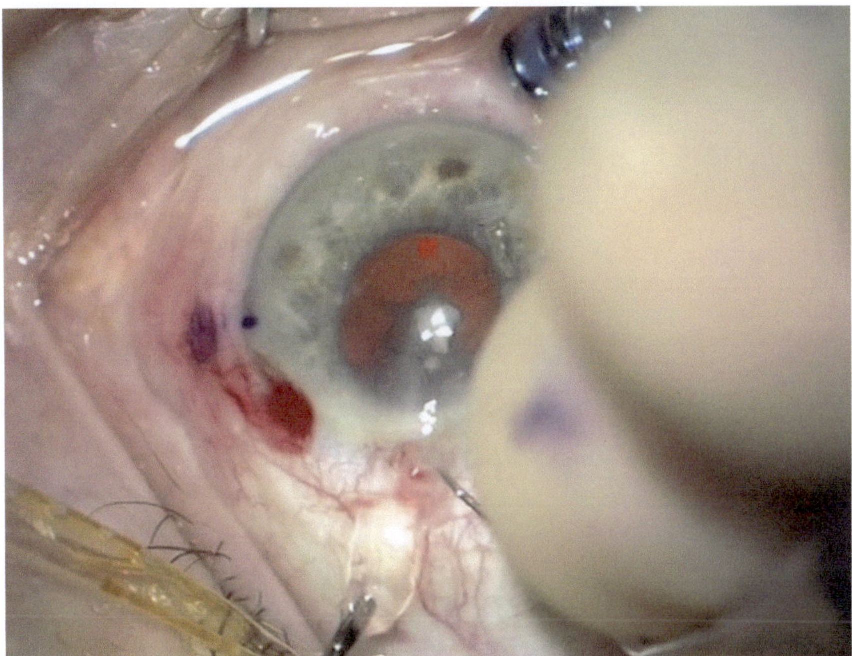

Fig. 19 Lifting of the anterior wound lip and passive outflow of residual capsular remnants

During IOL implantation care is taken that the two trailing haptics are positioned within the corneal wound, so that the two closed loops are easily threaded with the second, trimmed polypropylene suture. Threading of the second suture may also be performed before the folding procedure of the IOL. The two suture ends again are externalized with the FN 2 mm from the limbus at the contralateral side. Then, the IOL is positioned behind the iris. By pulling the four sutures, centration of the IOL can be achieved (Fig. 24). The suture ends are shortened now. As there is some mild tension applied to the sutures during the flanging maneuver, a conjunctival erosion does usually not occur with this approach. Instead, the flanges will slide into the external opening of the scleral tunnels and the conjunctiva and Tenon will cover the flanged sutures.

It is advisable to evacuate OVD if used during the previous steps. The port is removed, the wound hydrated and an intracameral antibiotic injected. Care is taken, that all flanges are covered by conjunctiva and all wounds are watertight. The pupil may be narrowed with a miotic agent.

No matter if we use flanged haptics or flanged sutures as our preferred fixation technique, grasping and externalisation is facilitated with the FN. Even in cases with poor visualisation due to corneal haze grasping is usually possible as optimal alignment of haptic or suture and needle are not mandatory. We can bring the end of the FN to an area allowing better visualisation and may grasp the haptic or suture end even at an odd angle before externalisation.

                                                    M. Amon et al.

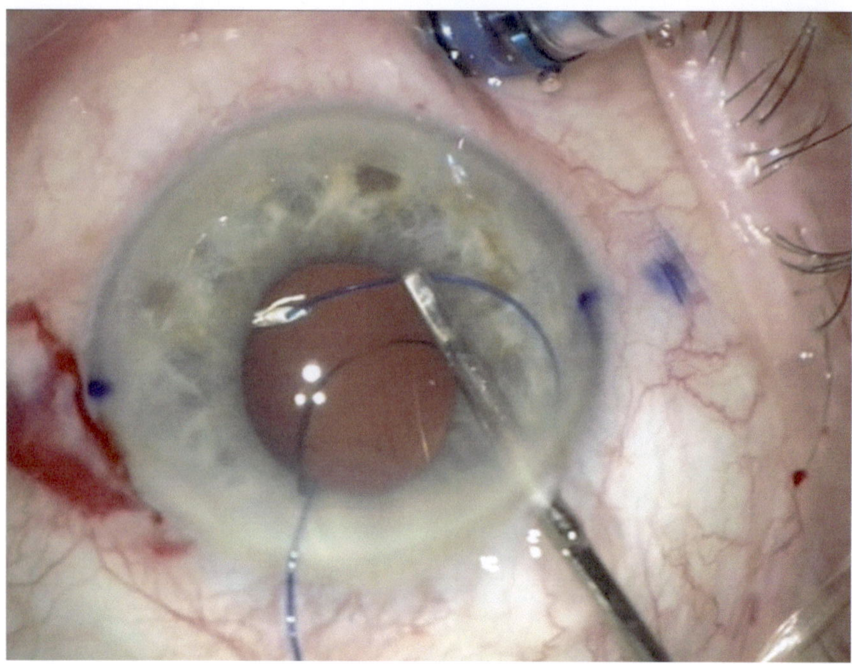

Fig. 20 Modified Yamane technique: the haptic-end (PVDF) is grasped by the FN before externalisation

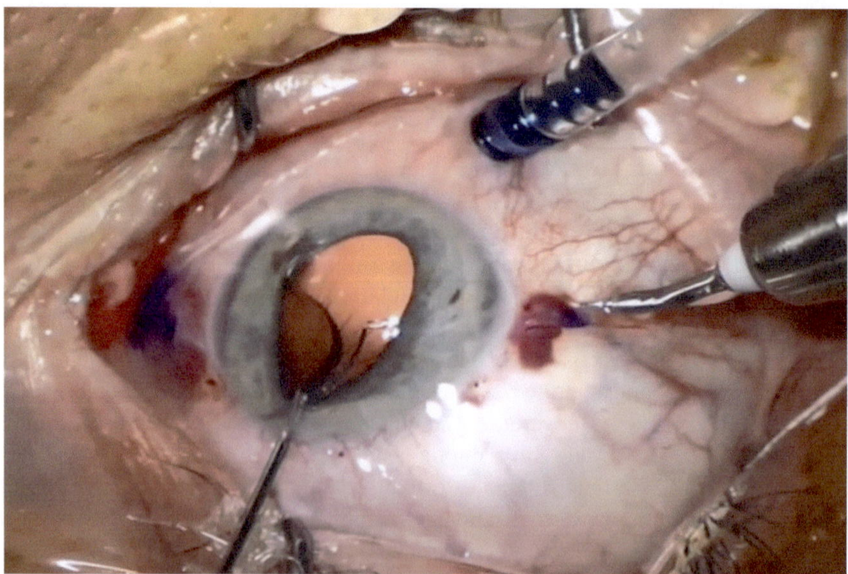

Fig. 21 Modified Yamane technique: the second haptic-end (PVDF) is grasped with the FN at a suboptimal angle

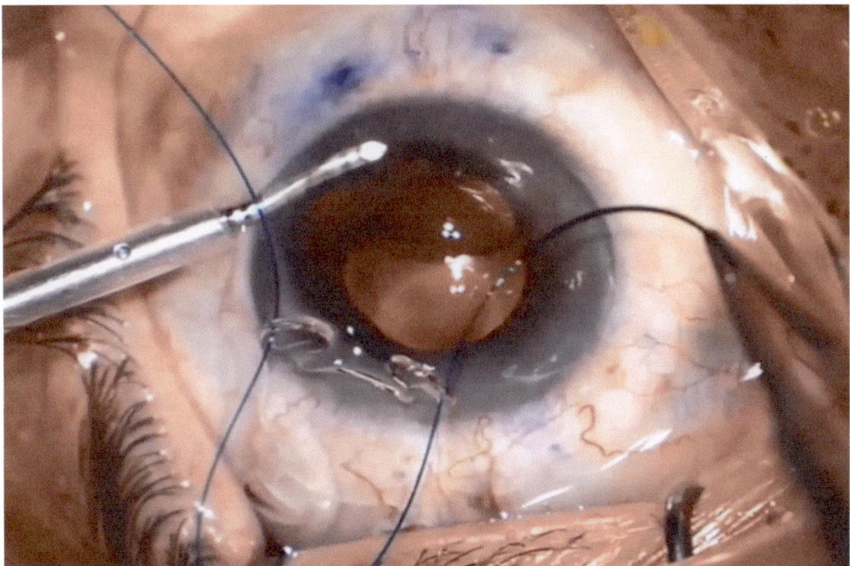

Fig. 22 Modified Canabrava technique: the 6-0 polypropylene suture is threaded through the first two closed loops of the IOL

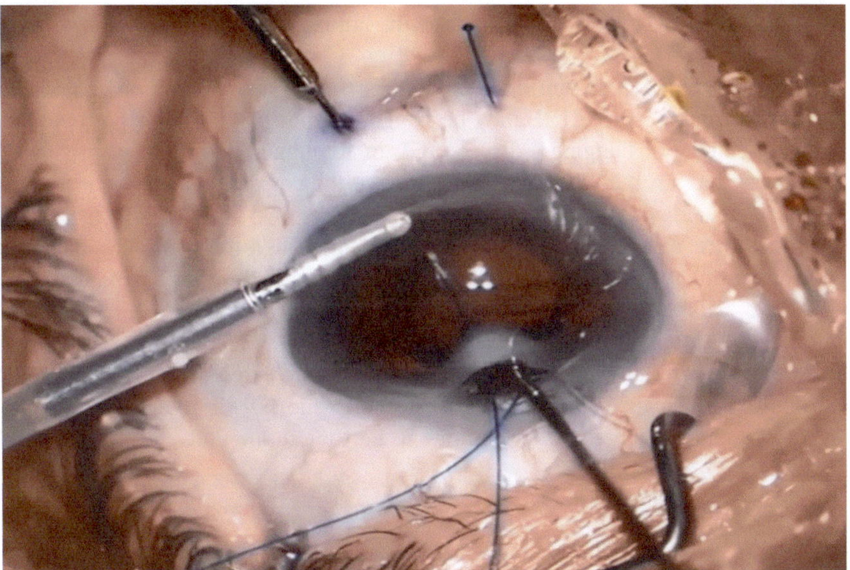

Fig. 23 Modified Canabrava technique: the second suture end is grasped and externalised with the FN after flanging of the first suture end

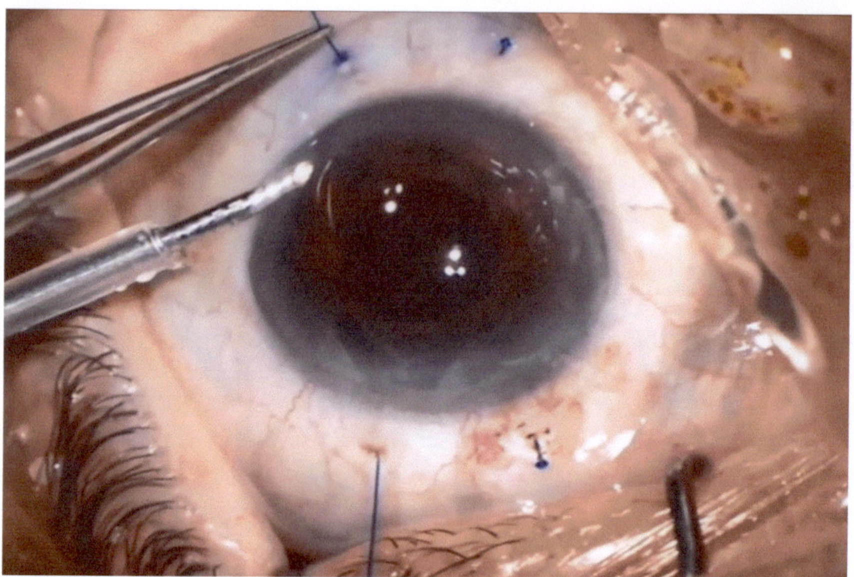

Fig. 24 Modified Canabrava technique: IOL centration with suture manipulation before flanging of all suture ends

In the key "takeaways" below we will summarize pros and cons of each technique.

In the rare situation of aniridia or large iris defects combined with aphakia an artificial iris and a 3-piece IOL may be flanged to the sclera. Pfeifer presented an elegant technique of flanging a 3-piece IOL in combination with an irisprosthesis [45]. Depending on the white to white distance the correct diameter of the artificial iris is created with a punch or with scissors. Then two holes are created within the artificial iris and the two haptics are threaded through the two holes. The iris/IOL compartment is folded and implanted into the anterior part of the eye. The two haptic-ends are externalized and flanged finally. In such a case I prefer a 4 point flanged suture fixation. I thread two 6-0 prolene sutures through an irisprosthesis together with an IOL with four closed loops and externalise the suture ends with the FN. Then the sandwich of irisprosthesis and IOL is folded with a folding forceps and implanted. After centration the four suture ends are trimmed and flanged.

Conclusion

For satisfying results in these complex cases of dislocated IOLs, capsular bags or of aphakia it is mandatory to find the best surgical procedure for each case. Sometimes decisions can only be made intraoperatively. This is caused by the fact that often only intraoperatively we can investigate the condition of the IOL, the condition of the capsular bag, the zonular support and the existence of a CTR. During this intraoperative inspection we have to find the most atraumatic approach, utilizing the best technique applicable. However, even with an optimized surgical approach in some cases we have to solve complications such as optic capture, conjunctival erosion, bleeding and decentration or tilt. Solutions for complications will be covered in the specific chapters and in the final "tips and tricks" and "question and answer" chapter.

All the flanging techniques are quite new and evolving. Therefore, there is a lack of randomized, prospective peer reviewed studies with enough power to find the single most favorable strategy for dislocated IOLs or for aphakia. However, we have to find the surgical approach we feel comfortable with most. This approach depends on our armamentarium of instruments and implants, on our surgical skills and the individual situation.

Chapter 7 gives a detailed overview of those instruments and implants which are important and helpful for the different flanging techniques in anterior segment surgery.

Key "Takeaways"

What Are the Pros of IOL Refixation Compared to IOL Exchange?

Pros IOL refixation:

- No main incision needed, no IOL exchange needed
- Only side ports and sometimes single scleral port needed
- Decentered IOL has proven to be biocompatible
- No biometry needed, biometrical result should not change with the same IOL
- Less surgical trauma, shorter surgical time
- Lower risk of luxation of lens-material to the posterior pole

Pros IOL exchange:

- Condition of luxated IOL does not matter
- Individual selection of the best IOL for scleral fixation
- Lens-material is removed completely in all cases
- Vitrectomy more controlled as no IOL is in the eye during vitrectomy
- Surgeons just needs skill for their best, single flanging technique

Flanging Haptics or Flanging Sutures for Perfect IOL Fixation?

Pros flanging two haptics:

- Only two scleral tunnels and only two flanges needed
- Shorter surgical time as with 4-point scleral suture fixation
- Easier IOL implantation with injector, no "suture confusion"
- Less biodegradiation of haptics as they are thicker than sutures
- Back-up IOL stock available as 3-piece IOLs are used for simple sulcus placement too

Pros double flanged sutures:

- Smaller flanges
- With 4 closed loop IOL a 4-point fixation potentially induces less tilt
- Exact length and exact position of scleral tunnels, if they are perpendicular
- Easier preparation of scleral tunnels
- Refixation of IOL/CTR- or IOL/capsule compartment is easier
- Plethora of options for fixation of IOLs, intraocular devices or ocular tissue

References

1. Yamane S, Sato S, Maruyama-Inoue M, Kadonosono K. Flanged intrascleral intraocular lens fixation with double-needle technique. Ophthalmology. 2017;124:1136–42.
2. Jakobsson G, Zetterberg M, Lundström M, et al. Late dislocation of in-the-bag and out-of-the bag intraocular lenses: ocular and surgical characteristics and time to lens repositioning. J Cataract Refract Surg. 2010;36:1637–44.
3. Clark A, Morlet N, Ng JQ, et al. Whole population trends in complications of cataract surgery over 22 years in Western Australia. Ophthalmology. 2011;118:1055–61.
4. Mönestam EI. Incidence of dislocation of intraocular lenses and pseudophakodonesis 10 years after cataract surgery. Ophthalmology. 2009;116:2315–20.
5. Lorente R, de Rojas V, Vazquez de Parga P, et al. Management of late spontaneous in-the-bag intraocular lens dislocation: retrospective analysis of 45 cases. J Cataract Refract Surg 2010;36:1270–1282.
6. Jehan FS, Mamalis N, Crandall AS. Spontaneous late dislocation of intraocular lens within the capsular bag in pseudoexfoliation patients. Ophthalmology. 2001;108:1727–31.
7. Gross JG, Kokame GT, Weinberg DV. Dislocated in-the-bag intraocular lens study group. In-the-bag intraocular lens dislocation. Am J Ophthalmol 2004;137:630–635.
8. Gimbel HV, Condon GP, Kohnen T, et al. Late in-the-bag intraocular lens dislocation: incidence, prevention, and management. J Cataract Refract Surg. 2005;31:2193–204.
9. Baumeister M, Bühren J, Kohnen T. Tilt and decentration of spherical and aspheric intraocular lenses: effect on higher-order aberrations. J Cataract Refract Surg. 2009;35:1006–12.
10. Oshika T, Sugita G, Miyata K, et al. Influence of tilt and decentration of scleral-sutured intraocular lens on ocular higher-order wavefront aberration. Br J Ophthalmol. 2007;91:185–8.
11. Taketani F, Matuura T, Yukawa E, Hara Y. Influence of intraocular lens tilt and decentration on wavefront aberrations. J Cataract Refract Surg. 2004;30:2158–62.

12. Grzybowski A, Markeviciute A, Zemaitiene R. A narrative review of intraocular lens opacifications: update 2020. Ann Transl Med. 2020;8:1547.

13. Fernández J, Sánchez-García A, Rodríguez-Vallejo M, Piñero DP. Systematic review of potential causes of intraocular lens opacification. Clin Experiment Ophthalmol. 2020;48:89–97.

14. Borkenstein AF, Borkenstein E-M. Analysis of YAG laser-induced damage in intraocular lenses: characterization of optical and surface properties of YAG shots. Ophthalmic Res. 2021;64:417–31.

15. Abela-Formanek C, Amon M, Schild G, et al. Uveal and capsular biocompatibility of hydrophilic acrylic, hydrophobic acrylic, and silicone intraocular lenses. J Cataract Refract Surg. 2002;28:50–61.

16. Özyol P, Özyol E, Karel F. Biocompatibility of intraocular lenses. Turk J Ophthalmol. 2017;47:221–5.

17. Dhital A, Spalton DJ, Goyal S, Werner L. Calcification in hydrophilic intraocular lenses associated with injection of intraocular gas. Am J Ophthalmol. 2012;153:1154-60.e1.

18. Grzybowski A, Zemaitiene R, Markeviciute A, Tuuminen R. Should we abandon hydrophilic intraocular lenses? Am J Ophthalmol. 2022;237:139–45.

19. Marcovich AL, Tandogan T, Bareket M, et al. Opacification of hydrophilic intraocular lenses associated with vitrectomy and injection of intraocular gas. BMJ Open Ophthalmol. 2018;3: e000157.

20. Hu J, Sella R, Afshari NA. Dysphotopsia: a multifaceted optic phenomenon. Curr Opin Ophthalmol. 2018;29:61–8.

21. Bonsemeyer MK, Becker E, Liekfeld A. Dysphotopsia and functional quality of vision after implantation of an intraocular lens with a 7.0 mm optic and plate haptic design. J Cataract Refract Surg 2022;48:75–82.

22. Masket S, Fram NR. Pseudophakic dysphotopsia: review of incidence, cause, and treatment of positive and negative dysphotopsia. Ophthalmology. 2021;128:e195–205.

23. Roop RP. Modified Scharioth's technique of scleral fixation of intraocular lens. Indian J Ophthalmol. 2017;65:1264–5.

24. Canabrava S, Andrade N Jr, Henriques PR. Scleral fixation of a 4-eyelet foldable intraocular lens in patients with aphakia using a 4-flanged technique. J Cataract Refract Surg. 2021;47:265–9.

25. Assia EI, Wong JXH. Adjustable 6-0 polypropylene flanged technique for scleral fixation, part 2: repositioning of subluxated IOLs. J Cataract Refract Surg. 2020;46:1392–6.

26. Auffarth GU, Beischel CJ, Wesendahl TA, Apple DJ. Soemmerring-Ring-Bildung nach Kataraktoperation und HKL-Implantation in menschlichen Autopsieaugen. In: 9. Kongreß der Deutschsprachigen Gesellschaft für Intraokularlinsen Implantation. Berlin: Springer; 1996. p. 408–413.

27. Rahimi M, Azimi A, Hosseinzadeh M. Intraocular lens calcification: clinico-pathological report of two cases and literature review. J Ophthalmic Vis Res. 2018;13:195–9.

28. Lavin M, Jagger J. Pathogenesis of pupillary capture after posterior chamber intraocular lens implantation. Br J Ophthalmol. 1986;70:886–9.

29. Heng LZ, Sandhu R, Snead DRJ, et al. Clinicopathologic correlation of lens epithelial metaplasia and late intraocular lens dislocation after repair of retinal detachment. JAMA Ophthalmol. 2016;134:827–830. Available at: Accessed 28 Nov 2022.

30. Culp C, Qu P, Jones J, et al. Clinical and histopathological findings in the dead bag syndrome. J Cataract Refract Surg. 2022;48:177–84.

31. Amon M, Bernhart C, Geitzenauer W, Kahraman G. The forceps-needle: combining needle and grasping functions in a single instrument. J Cataract Refract Surg. 2021;47:123–6.

32. Madanagopalan VG, Sen P, Baskaran P. Scleral-fixated intraocular lenses. TNOA J Ophthalmic Sci Res 2018;56:237. Available at: Accessed 28 Nov 2022.

33. Barber FA, Herbert MA, Beavis RC, Barrera OF. Suture anchor materials, eyelets, and designs: update 2008. Arthroscopy. 2008;24:859–67.

34. Ton Y, Naftali M, Lapid-Gortzak R, Assia EI. Management of subluxated capsular bag-fixated intraocular lenses using a capsular anchor. J Cataract Refract Surg. 2016;42:653–8.

35. Tsao SW, Holz HA. Iris mattress suture: a technique for sectoral iris defect repair. Br J Ophthalmol. 2015;99:305–7.
36. Lian RR, Siepser SB, Afshari NA. Iris reconstruction suturing techniques. Curr Opin Ophthalmol. 2020;31:43–9.
37. Kramer BA, Hardten DR, Berdahl JP. Rotation characteristics of three toric monofocal intraocular lenses. Clin Ophthalmol. 2020;14:4379–84.
38. Potvin R, Kramer BA, Hardten DR, Berdahl JP. Toric intraocular lens orientation and residual refractive astigmatism: an analysis. Clin Ophthalmol. 2016;10:1829–36.
39. Silva N, Ferreira A, Ferreira N, et al. Intrascleral knotless zigzag suture fixation of four-haptic hydrophilic acrylic foldable IOL: clinical outcomes. Clin Ophthalmol. 2022;16:33–41.
40. Mamalis N. Explantation of intraocular lenses. Curr Opin Ophthalmol. 2000;11:289–95.
41. Fernández-Buenaga R, Alio JL, Muñoz-Negrete FJ, et al. Causes of IOL explantation in Spain. Eur J Ophthalmol. 2012;22:762–8.
42. Neuhann T, Yildirim TM, Son H-S, et al. Reasons for explantation, demographics, and material analysis of 200 intraocular lens explants. J Cataract Refract Surg. 2020;46:20–6.
43. Mamalis N, Crandall AS, Pulsipher MW, et al. Intraocular lens explantation and exchange. A review of lens styles, clinical indications, clinical results, and visual outcome. J Cataract Refract Surg 1991;17:811–818.
44. Wilczyński M, Wilczyńska O, Omulecki W. Analysis of causes of intraocular lens explantations in the material of Department of Ophthalmology, Medical University of Lodz. Klin Oczna. 2009;111:21–5.
45. Pfeifer V, Marzidovšek M, Marzidovšek ZL. Artificial Iris Implantation: overview of surgical techniques. In: Cataract surgery. 2022. p. 321–338. Available at: Accessed 28 Nov 2022.

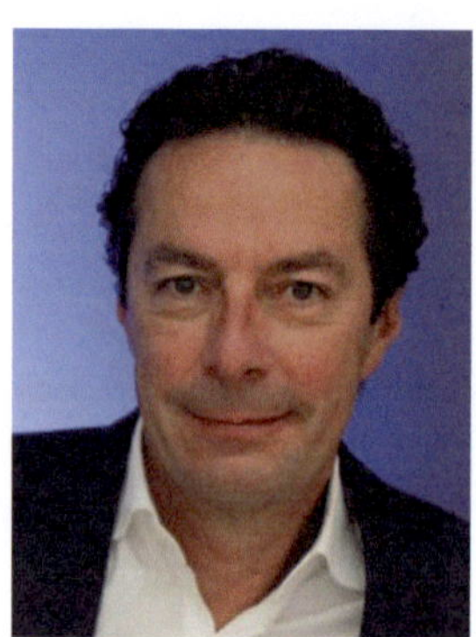

Michael Amon Chair of ophthalmology, Sigmund Freud Medical University Vienna; Head of eye-department, Academic Teaching Hospital Vienna; Johannes von Gott Platz 1, 1020 Wien.

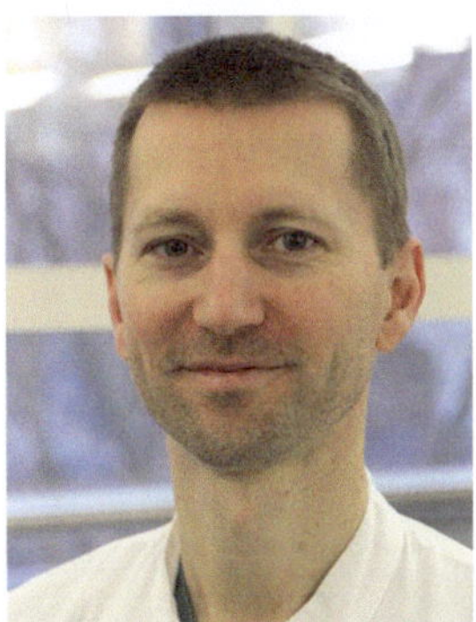

Wolfgang Geitzenauer Sigmund Freud Medical University Vienna; Academic Teaching Hospital Vienna; Johannes von Gott Platz 1, 1020 Wien.

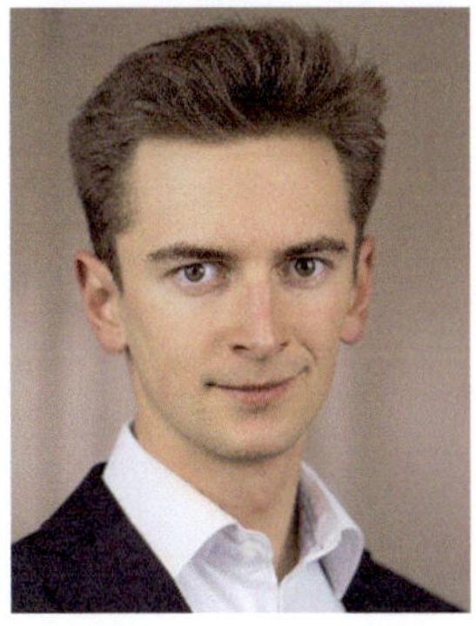

Konstantin Seiller-Tarbuk is an ophthalmologist from Vienna. Having studied at the Medical University of Vienna he is currently finishing his residency at the Hospital of St. John of God. In addition to his clinical work, Konstantin has actively engaged in teaching lessons and practical courses, sharing his knowledge and expertise with physicians, medical students and nursing professionals for many years. Additionally, he brings a unique and innovative perspective as a young doctor. In combination with his knowledge in video and photo editing, he is a valuable contributor to the book chapter, bringing insights and practical knowledge to the table.

Utilizing Optimized Instruments and Implants

Wolfgang Geitzenauer, Konstantin Seiller-Tarbuk, and Michael Amon

Abstract

The best surgical plan to restore the vision of a patient in need of an IOL exchange, IOL re-fixation or a secondary IOL will not be successful without the specific instruments and implants needed for each technique available. While a detailed description of each author's specific approach is given in the corresponding chapter, we aim to provide a brief overview of some instruments we found helpful in our everyday practice. Knowing that there are limitations in regional availability of both instruments and lens implants we do not mean our list of mentioned devices to be exhaustive. Our goal is to merely present a helpful selection of what we know has worked in our experience.

Keywords

Flanging technique · Instruments · IOL · Forceps-needle

Infusion

Anterior chamber maintainers have been used widely in ophthalmic surgery in the past. Phacoemulsification and other procedures continuously improved over time, including smaller incision sizes, better intraocular pressure control via phaco machines and reduced stress of intraocular tissue due to better IOL characteristics. Hence, the need for anterior chamber maintainers has declined over the years and

Supplementary Information The online version contains supplementary material available at https://doi.org/10.1007/978-3-031-32855-8_7.

W. Geitzenauer (✉) · K. Seiller-Tarbuk · M. Amon
Academic Teaching Hospital of St. John, Vienna, Austria
e-mail: wolfgang.geitzenauer@bbwien.at

is nowadays not that common in routine cases as it was in the past. Nevertheless, these instruments become valuable tools when dealing with more complex cases or in IOL exchange procedures.

Anterior chamber maintainers (Fig. 1) are available in different gauge sizes and allow improved stability of the intraocular pressure gradient between the anterior and the posterior chamber. While the presence of a scleral port infusion via the pars plana can help to keep a subluxated IOL from further displacement posteriorly during the steps of explantation, a stable anterior chamber greatly facilitates steps involving manipulation of tissue and handling instruments from anteriorly. Particularly, when placing instruments through the rigid sclera the presence of an anterior chamber maintainer may aid in the wound construction and may add to the pressure stability of the globe. The risk of an intraocular hemorrhage due to partial loss of pressure when introducing a needle or a trocar into the globe may be significantly reduced as well. A potential disadvantage is the crowding in the anterior chamber due to the presence of an additional instrument, depending on the gauge size. Further potential disadvantages include reduced visibility behind an AC maintainer. During IOL or suture manipulation an AC maintainer might come in the way and make the maneuvers more complex than without it.

Trocar-assisted posterior infusion via the pars plana is another way of facilitating an IOL exchange procedure (Fig. 1). Not only becomes the posterior access helpful in controlling the pressure gradient during a particular maneuver when needed, it is also an excellent opportunity to carry out an anterior vitrectomy more efficiently. When both an AC maintainer and a pars plana trocar are available, switching the access for the vitrectomy and infusion will help in the complete removal of potential vitreous. Despite the advantages of the presence of a scleral

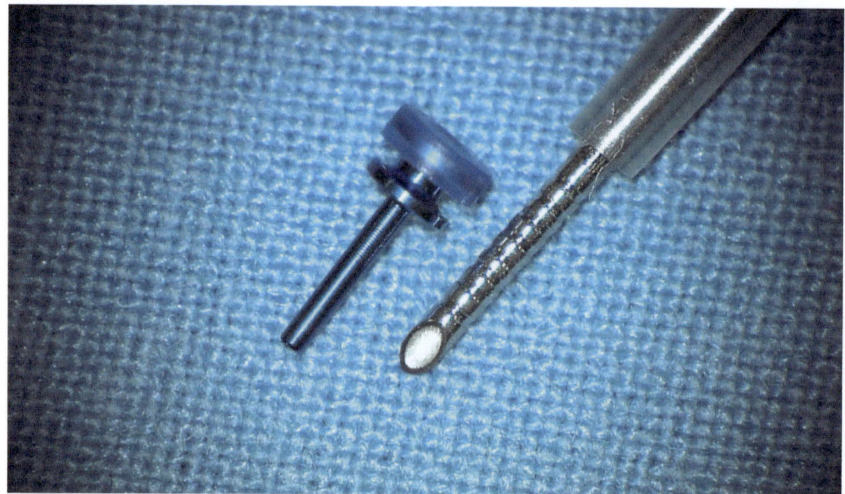

Fig. 1 25 gauge scleral port (left) compared to a 20 gauge anterior chamber maintainer (right). Smaller anterior chamber maintainers are available

port there is a higher risk of bleeding. Depending on the proximity of a scleral port and the target area for needle or suture placement during later stages of the procedure the visibility might become impaired.

Pars-plana trocar	Anterior chamber maintainer
+ Vitrectomy more sufficient + Size irrelevant (23-gauge, 25-gauge, 27-gauge) − Higher risk of bleeding	+ No need for scleral port − Anterior chamber more crowded − Size (20-gauge, 23-gauge, 25-gauge) − Corneal warping

Marking

Marking the globe for ideal positioning of flanges is one of the key aspects of successful scleral fixation of an IOL. Keeping the flange positions at an angle of exactly 180° helps to keep the IOL centered. The ideal orientation of the axis is yet to be determined. However, in many cases the 3 and 9 o'clock positions will be selected as they were initially described and became a common approach by many surgeons. 2:30 and 8:30 o'clock positions may be used alternatively to avoid the risk of affecting the anterior ciliary arteries or long ciliary nerves although no higher risk of damage to these structures has been reported yet.

Apart from adhering to the 180° angle an identical distance from the limbus to the transconjunctival entry site as well as an identical length of the scleral tunnel are equally important to reduce the risk of IOL decentration or tilt. A commonly used distance is 2 mm posterior from the limbus although some surgeons favor 2.5 mm in order to reduce the risk of potential damage to the ciliary body. Several instruments facilitate the marking of entry sites, including measuring rings (e.g., Mendez degree marker (Fig. 2), Storz Ophthalmic Instruments, USA) or calipers. Careful preoperative planning of instrument access becomes even more important when planning to use a toric IOL for scleral fixation.

Yamane Double-Needle Stabilizer

The Yamane Double-needle Stabilizer (Fig. 3) is an instrument that simplifies the identification of the sclerotomy sites without the need of prior marking. Additionally, it provides control over the angles of insertion when creating the scleral tunnels. This ring-shaped instrument allows for good fixation of the eye due to its shape and toothed base. It provides two grooved platforms located 180° apart at an intended distance of 2 mm from the limbus, eliminating the need for axis markers, calipers or ink. The two platforms facilitate creating reproducible scleral tunnels and thus minimize stress on IOL haptics once tucked in. These allow passing the needle through the instrument and inserting the needle at a predefined angle of 20° to the corneal limbus and 10° to the surface of the iris.

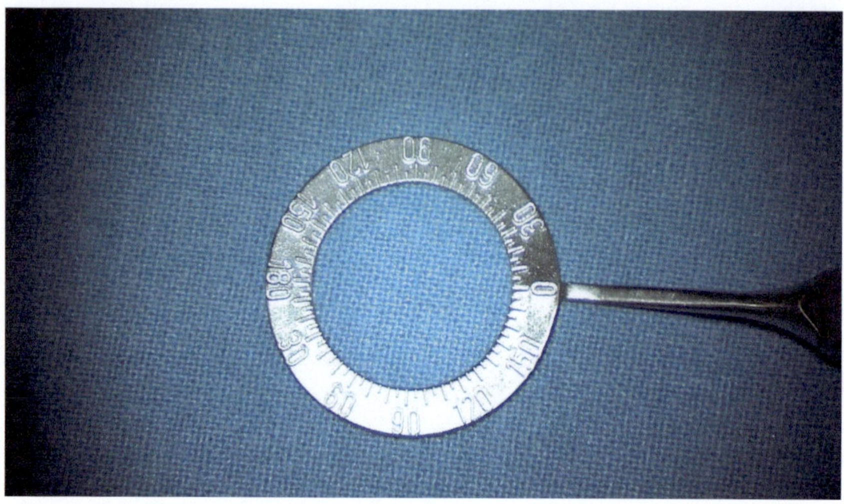

Fig. 2 Mendez degree marker (Storz Ophthalmic Instruments)

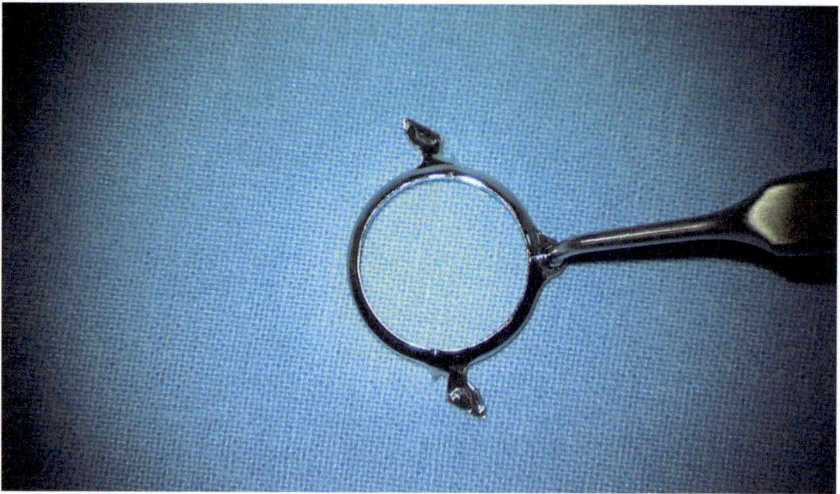

Fig. 3 Yamane double-needle stabilizer (Geuder)

One limitation of this instrument is its fixed diameter. This might or might not fit well to the globe depending on its corneal diameter and axial length. Hence, the final entry sites in the sclera might not be 2 mm away from the limbus. Alternatively, using calipers allows the exact measurement of the anticipated distance from the limbus regardless of the corneal diameter.

Tools for Externalization of Haptics

Thin-Walled Needles

The emphasis lies on 'thin-walled' as standard needles either have a lumen diameter of 0.14 mm (30 gauge) or 0.21 mm (27 gauge) (Figs. 4, 5 and 6). Haptics of commonly used 3-piece IOLs (0.14 to 0.17 mm) are too thick to be fed into the lumen of a conventional 30 gauge needle. They can be used in conjunction with 27-gauge needles, however, as their outer diameter is significantly greater (0.40 mm) than those of a 30-gauge needle the risk of hypotony and flange perforation through the thicker scleral tunnel is higher [16, 17]. In general, the inner diameter of needles of a specific gauge size seems to vary significantly between manufacturers.

One manufacturer of a needle available unifies the characteristics that facilitate successful externalization of haptics when using a hollow needle approach is TSK Laboratories (Tochigi, Japan). They produce a 30-gauge hypodermic needle suitable for feeding haptics of 3-piece IOLs. Although some specifications of diameter and lumen sizes are reported in the literature, the manufacturer did not reveal those to the authors upon e-mail request for commercial reasons.

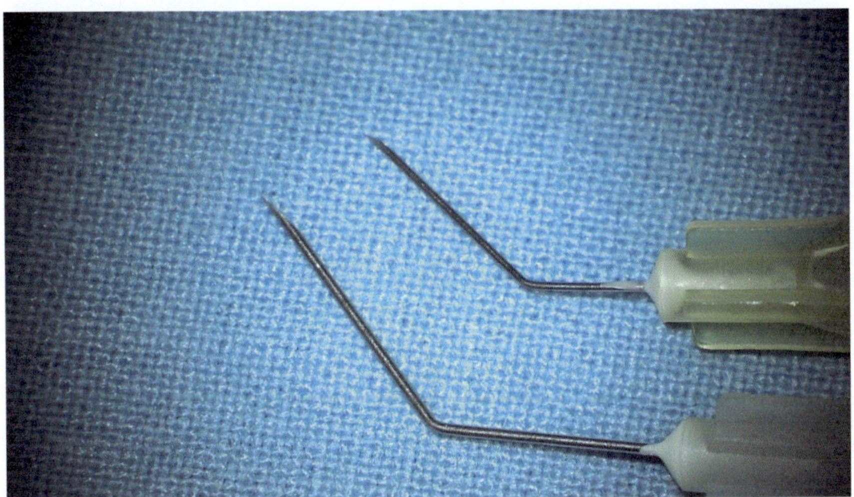

Fig. 4 Comparison of a 30 gauge (top) and a 27 gauge (bottom) hypodermic needle (both conventional) after bending with a needle-holder

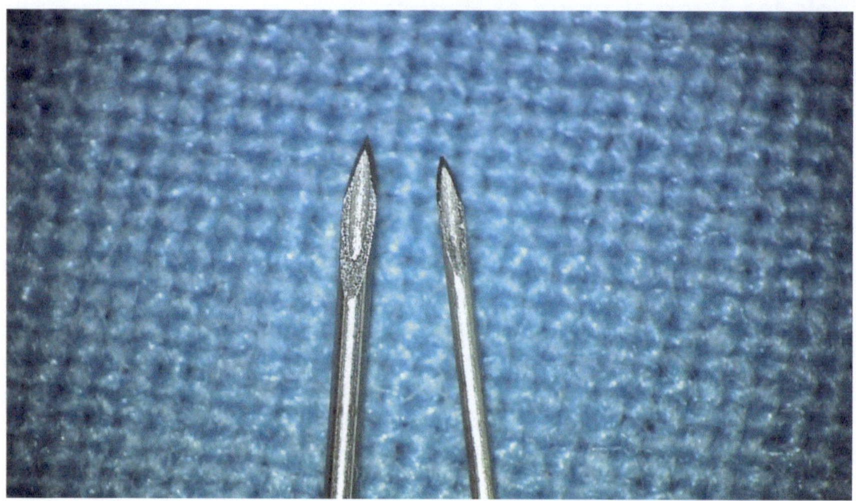

Fig. 5 Comparison of a 27 gauge (left) and a 30 gauge (right) hypodermic needle (both conventional)

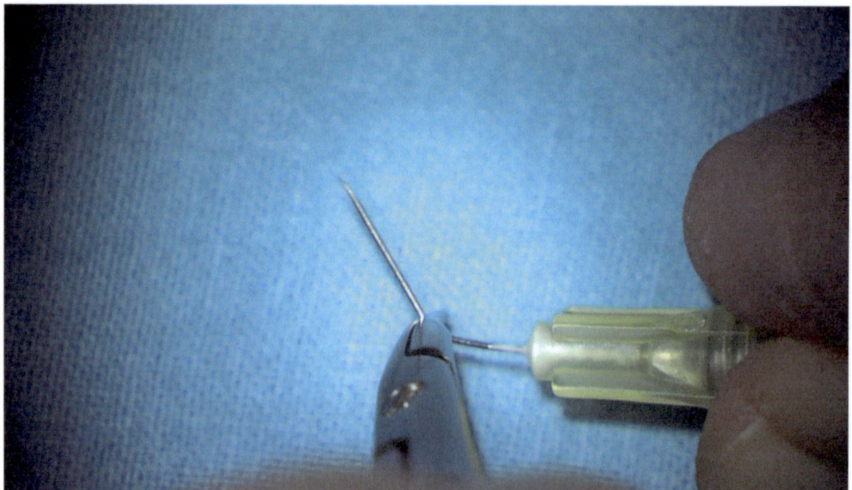

Fig. 6 Bending a 30 gauge hypodermic needle with a needle-holder

Amon Forceps-Needle

The Amon Forceps Needle [3] facilitates many steps of flanged intrascleral haptic- or suture fixation and can be especially useful in complicated cases (Figs. 7 and 8). It is intended to create access to the posterior chamber similar to a cannula to grasp IOL haptics, sutures or tissue at the same time. The main benefit is the simplification of grasping and externalizing of IOL haptics or sutures. There is no additional need for feeding the haptic or a thread into a thin-walled needle due to its grasping function.

The forceps-needle is currently available in a 27 gauge diameter as a reusable instrument. It is bent 145° and holds a blunt grasping forceps within the lumen of the needle. A standardized handpiece is used and provides ergonomic control.

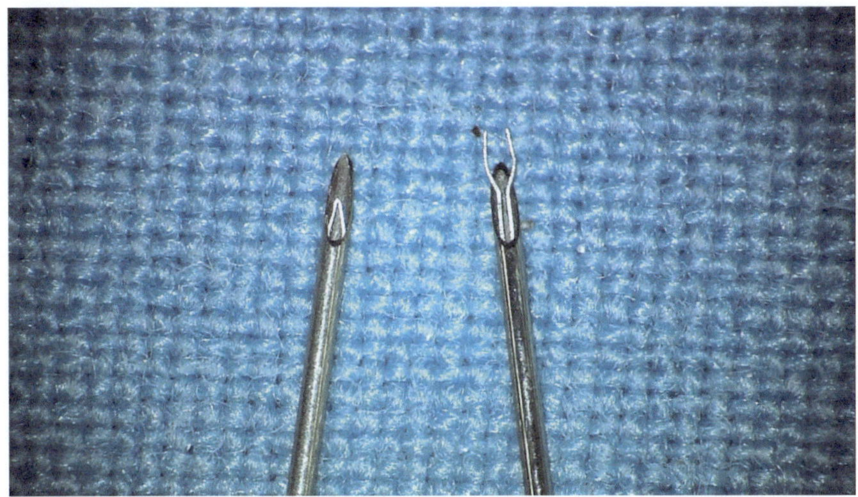

Fig. 7 Amon forceps-needle (Geuder), 27 gauge version. Left: forceps closed, Right: forceps open

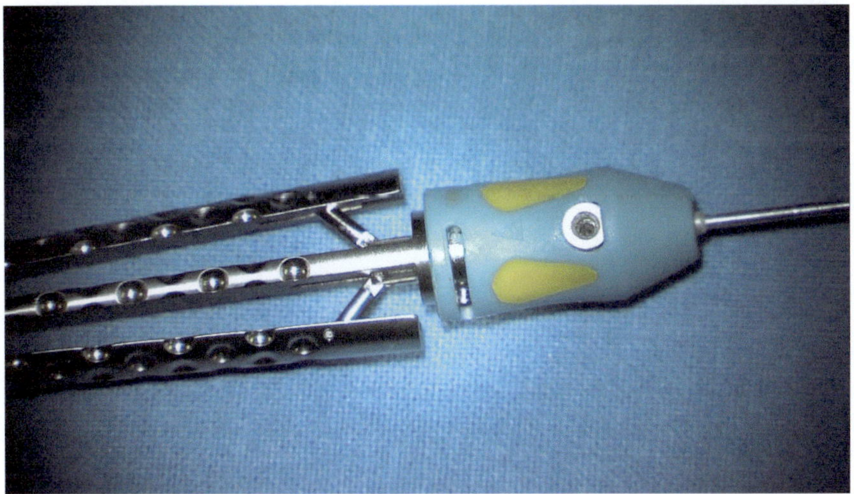

Fig. 8 Amon forceps-needle (Geuder), detail of handpiece mechanism (prototype of the disposable version)

Triggers in the handpiece control the forceps inside the sharp needle. The forceps is designed in a way that it retracts inside the needle when closed while holding the grasped object. In the near future, there will be a single use version available, as well as a 30 gauge size version.

Possible applications are: scleral fixation (e.g., Yamane technique, Canabrava technique, Scharioth technique, Gore-Tex glued IOL), fixation of capsular tension rings or capsular segments, iris fixation of IOLs, Gore-Tex and polypropylene sutures as well as refixation of undamaged closed loop IOLs and 3-piece IOLs.

A link to the video showing the instrument is available in the section "Electronic Supplementary Material".

Additional Instruments

Cautery

Disposable high or low temperature cautery (Fig. 9) is the method of choice to create a flanged tip at a haptic or suture end. Although other methods can be found in the literature [1] including an endolaser probe or a thermal ball tip cautery, low temperature cautery is regarded as the most practical and cost-effective approach and provides better control of the flange creation. Depending on the distance between the cautery tip and the haptic or suture end a more or less wide flange can be created. In respect to IOL haptics, the flange configuration also depends on the material used. By far, the vast majority of three-piece IOLs on the market come with haptics made of polymethylmethacrylate (PMMA). This material has proven ideal for its intended purpose for a long time. However, with the advances of techniques of intrascleral haptic fixation and the widespread use it has taken on, another material has gained interest in the ophthalmic community. Polyvinylidene fluoride (PVDF) has been used for IOL haptics for a long time. Cautery of haptics made of it seem to yield wider flanges [9]. Also, the distance of the holding forceps to the end of the held haptic or suture influences the flange configuration and its size. Caution is needed in order not to let the tip of the cautery touch the haptic/suture end as it might stick to it or form the flange in a way left unsuitable for fixation.

Holding Forceps

A wide range of intraocular holding forceps is available for handling of IOL haptics while feeding it into a transscleral needle (Fig. 10). Depending on personal preference and anatomical needs (e.g., approach from nasally in patients with a prominent nose) straight or bent models can be used, e.g. the Scharioth IOL Scleral Fixation straight and curved forceps, (*D.O.R.C., Zuidland, The Netherlands*).

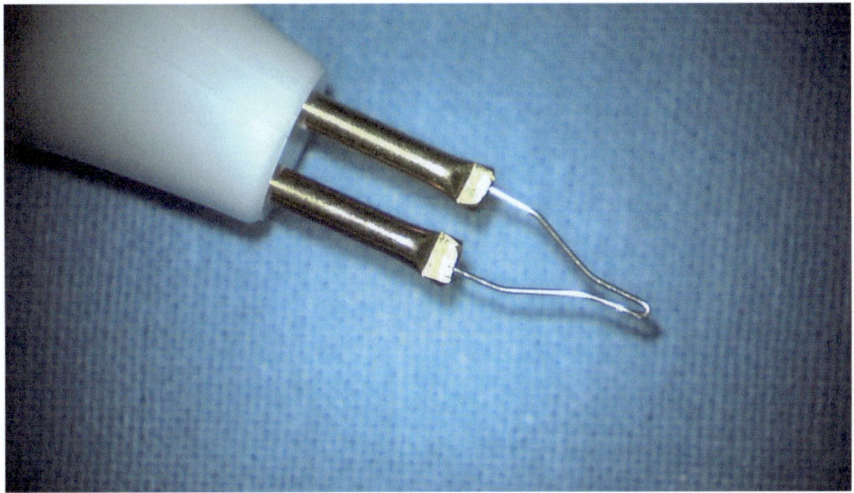

Fig. 9 Low-temperature cautery

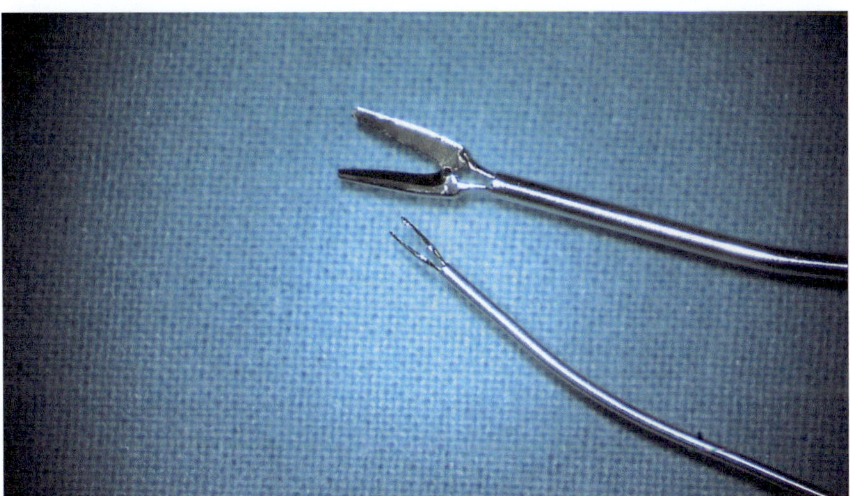

Fig. 10 Snyder/Osher IOL explantation set (Geuder)

Another factor to take into consideration is the angle while grasping, whether horizontal or vertical modes of action are better suited. Also, some forceps seem to make it less smooth to enter or exit the eye through a standard paracentesis due to their design features (e.g., edges getting caught at the inner anterior lip of the wound). Gripping vitreoretinal forceps are helpful especially if IOL recovery from the posterior segment is needed (Fig. 11).

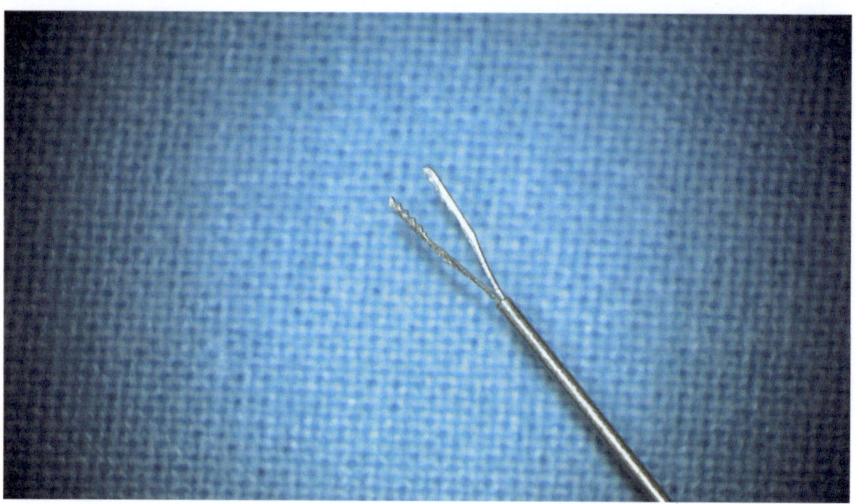

Fig. 11 25 gauge vitreoretinal forceps

Sutures

A variety of different suture materials in a range of diameters is readily available. There is no consensus which suture is generally best suited for scleral fixation and the debate is continuing. Polypropylene (*Prolene*®, Ethicon/Johnson & Johnson Surgical Technologies) and Polytetrafluoroethylene (Gore-Tex®, *Gore & Associates Inc.*) are the two most common used materials currently.

Many surgeons prefer 6-0 monofilament polypropylene sutures and argue that the tensile strength combined with their relative flexibility to handle them intraocularly make them the best compromise for IOL fixation. In addition, the better biodegradation rate compared to smaller diameters make it less susceptible to possible secondary IOL dislocation in the future. Widespread use has taken on after new techniques were published, e.g. the Four-Flanged Intrascleral Intraocular Lens Fixation Technique by Canabrava et al. [6]. 10-0 polypropylene sutures have been used for intrascleral haptic fixation but reports show significant breakage rates in the follow-up period over a mean of 50 months [14, 15].

Multiple variables influence the breaking strength of sutures apart from its gauge size. Additionally, the amount of suture length cauterized (e.g. 0.5 or 1.0 mm) and the relation of sclerotomy to suture gauge do matter. Furthermore, flange size decreased with smaller-gauge sutures and smaller gauges have lower pull-through forces (Fig. 12).

Polytetrafluoroethylene (Gore-Tex®) sutures, traditionally used in the 7-0 dimension, are another option, though their use is off-label. Compared to 5-0 to 7-0 polypropylene they have to be brought into the eye by long needle passes through the anterior chamber and cannot be tucked into lumen of needles. This also applies to traditionally used 10-0 polypropylene sutures for refixation of IOLs.

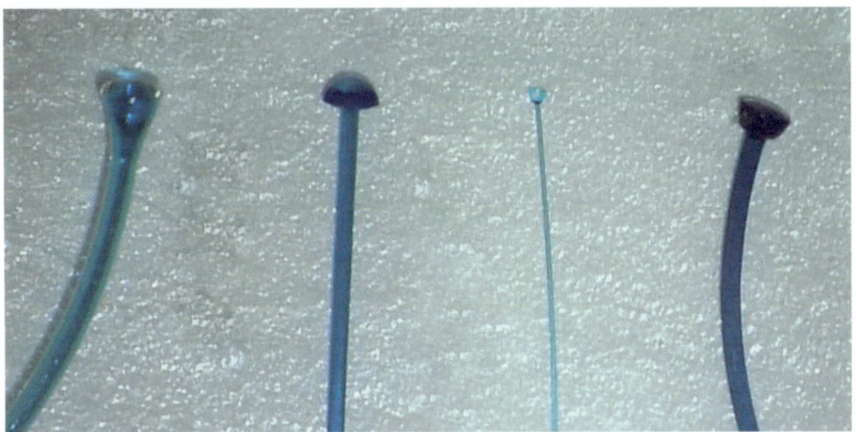

Fig. 12 Comparison of flanges yielded after application of low-temperature cautery. From left to right: PMMA haptic of a AR40e IOL (Johnson & Johnson), 6-0 polypropylene suture, 10-0 polypropylene suture, PVDF haptic of an Avansee IOL (Kowa)

While 8-0 polypropylene sutures and 0.5 mm flanges should provide sufficient long-term stability, 1.0-mm flanges using 5-0 to 7-0 polypropylene and 27- to 30-gauge sclerotomies are recommended.

IOL Selection

The design and type of the IOL will mainly influence the decision-making process as already described in detail in previous chapters. The following section aims to create a brief overview of common IOL models used for intrascleral haptic fixation.

IOLs for Flanged Haptic Fixation

Three Piece IOLs

Haptic Materials

The most common materials used for IOL haptics are polymethylmethacrylate (PMMA), polyamide, polypropylene and polyvinylidene fluoride (PVDF). Nowadays, mainly PMMA and PVDF are used by manufacturers. Regarding stability against deformation the haptic materials can be divided into two groups: more deformable IOL haptics (PMMA, polyamide, polypropylene) and less deformable IOL haptics (PVDF). All these materials can be used for flanged intrascleral haptic fixation. PVDF haptics make intraocular maneuvering easier and less susceptible to breakage due to their flexibility. A study investigating biomechanical stability

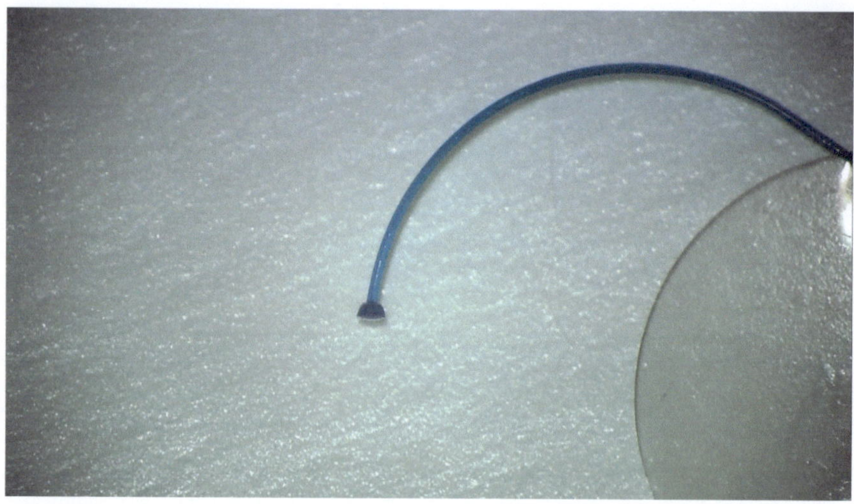

Fig. 13 PVDF haptic of an Avansee Preset PU6A (Kowa) IOL after applying low-temperature cautery

found that the force needed to dislocate the haptics from the IOL was higher in an IOL with PVDF than in a different model with PMMA haptics [9]. On the other hand, the increased rigidity of PVDF haptics results in higher resistance against manipulation making feeding the trailing haptic into the lumen of the needle more difficult. Low heat cautery applied to PVDF seems to yield a flange shape (mushroom style) better suited for transscleral fixation than to PMMA (cone shaped) (Figs. 12, 13 and 14).

Polymethylmethacrylate (PMMA)
+ widely available

− susceptible for kinking

− susceptible for breaking

Polyvinylidene Fluoride (PVDF)
+ less deformable

+ high memory

+ better flange configuration (mushroom shaped)

The following list is merely a selection of IOLs that have been used for flanged intrascleral fixation and is not meant to be complete. Due to regional and national differences in availability and health authority clearance we aim to highlight a few models we believe are often used and have been mentioned in some reports about

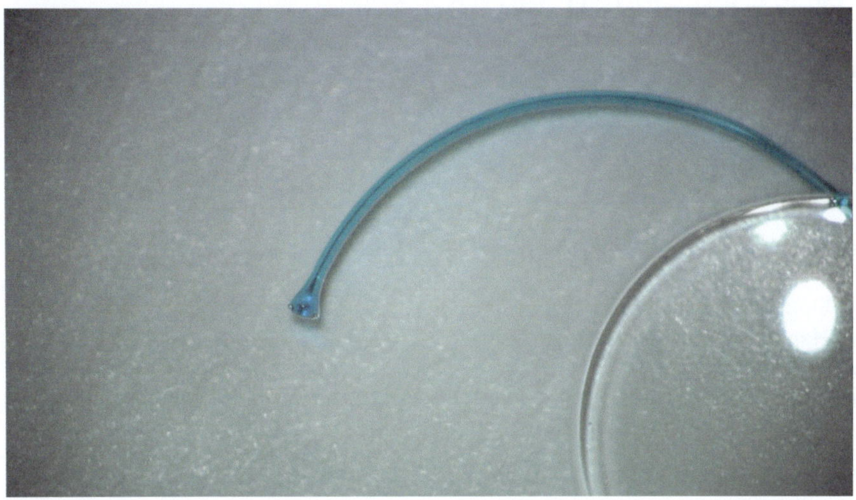

Fig. 14 PMMA haptic of a Johnson & Johnson SENSAR AR40e IOL after applying low-temperature cautery

intrascleral fixation. A complete list was not considered to be feasible as the sheer number of IOLs on the market is exhaustive (https://iolcon.org/).

Alcon AcrySof MA60MA and MA60AC

- Optic material: acrylic
- Haptic material: PMMA
- −5.0 to +30.0 D
- monofocal

Zeiss CT LUCIA 202/602

- Optic material: acrylic
- Haptic material: PVDF
- +4.0 to +34.0 D
- monofocal, sphere (202) or asphere (602)

Bausch and Lomb EYE-Cee

- Optic material: acrylic
- Haptic material: PMMA
- +10.0 to +28.0 D
- monofocal, sphere

Millenium Biomedical SAL 300A/AC

- Optic material: acrylic
- Haptic material: PMMA
- 0.0 to 30.0 D
- monofocal, asphere

Johnson & Johnson SENSAR AR40e/E/M

- Optic material: acrylic
- Haptic material: PMMA
- -10.0 to $+30.0$ D
- monofocal, sphere

Bausch & Lomb SofPort LI61AOR

- Optic material: silcone
- Haptic material: PMMA
- 0.0 to $+34.0$ D
- monofocal, asphere

Kowa AvanseePreset PU6A/S and PN6A/S

- Optic material: acrylic
- Haptic material: PVDF
- $+6.0$ to $+26.0$
- monofocal, asphere
- clear (PU6A/S) or yellow (PN6A/S)

IOLs for Suture Fixation

The vast majority of IOLs can be used for suture fixation. Those with preexisting loops or holes in its haptics facilitate the surgical technique significantly.

Single-piece IOLs without those design characteristics can be suture fixated as well using a piercing technique (e.g., the Piercing Flanged Technique by Carhalho et al. (*Piercing Flanged Technique Durval Carvalho Jr -Winner World Webinar Cataract and Refractive Surgery*, 2021)). Multifocal or toric monofocal IOLs usually do not feature loops or holes. Hence, they would have to be replaced by three-piece IOLs losing their premium characteristics if they cannot be re-fixated in cases such as loss of zonular support.

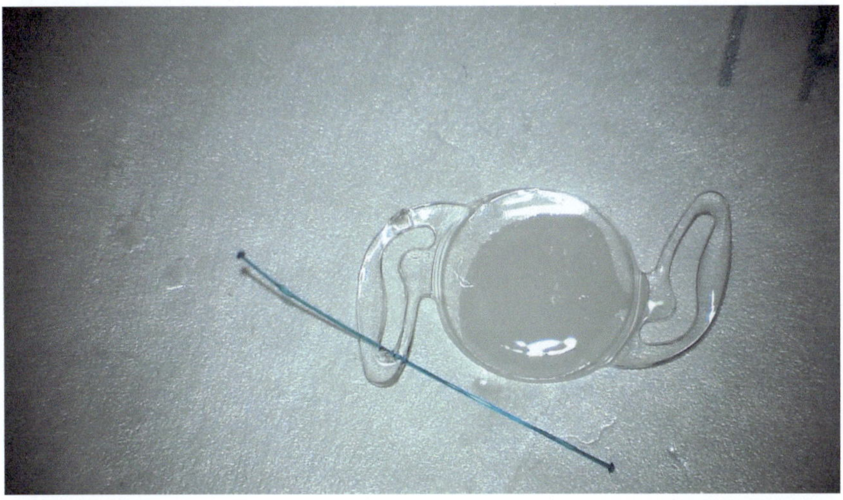

Fig. 15 RAO600C IOL (Rayner) with haptics pierced using a 6-0 polypropylene suture (both ends flanged)

Although 3-piece IOLs can be sutured to the sclera without flanging [2], the advent of recent techniques described above make them nowadays obsolete in most cases.

The market offers a wide variety of IOLs with closed loops, closed haptics or modified plate haptics. All of them offer the chance to be fixated to the sclera using sutures. Models with 4 loops or haptics have the potential to improve centration and distribution of holding forces and carry less risk of IOL tilt when using 4-point fixation. IOLs with closed loops or modified plate haptics allow refixation of the IOL by threading a suture through the hole serving as an eyelet. Techniques have been described for 2-point fixation of closed loop IOLs in the past [10] and offer a technically less demanding way to fixate and center such lenses (Fig. 15). Four-point IOL fixation is sometimes associated with an easier learning curve, since it omits the difficult step of insertion of the trailing haptic. Although tilt and decentration being one of its documented complications, various four-point fixation techniques have been shown to yield better stability and prevent tilt when compared with other techniques. [5, 10, 13] (Fig. 16).

Other IOL Designs

Some IOL manufacturers provide eyelets in their design, anticipating the potential need for secondary support using sutures at a later stage (e.g. Bausch & Lomb enVista, Oculentis Femtis, SIFI Mini, VSY Acriva, Zeiss AT LISA).

In addition to standard monofocal IOLs a variety of multifocal and extended range of vision IOL designs with four closed loops are available on the market.

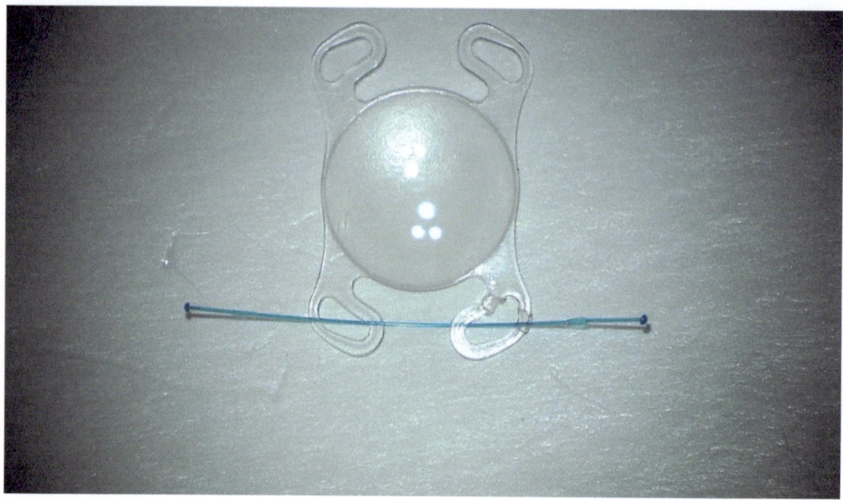

Fig. 16 Akreos IOL (Bausch & Lomb) with double-flanged 6-0 polypropylene suture

Also, IOLs that are specifically designed to be placed in the ciliary sulcus (Cristalens Reverso, 1stQ, Rayner Sulcoflex) may be sutured using the piercing flanged technique and possible rotation prevented (Fig. 17) [8]. Although rare, rotation of a toric add-on IOL might occur. Should the rotation back to the original position as an initial step not be sufficient then suture-fixation is a valuable tool to keep the IOL in the desired position.

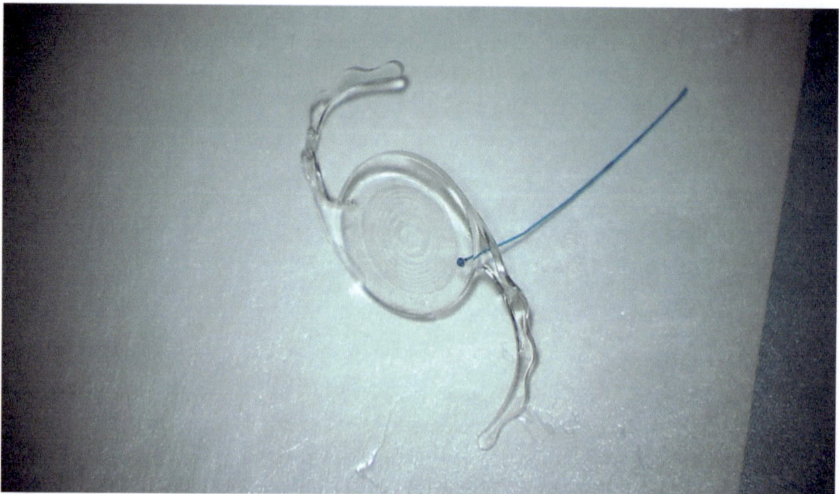

Fig. 17 Sulcoflex Toric IOL (Rayner) shown after piercing the haptic-optic junction with a 6-0 polypropylene suture and flanging with low-temperature cautery

Md tech (Casoria, Italy) is the manufacturer of a single piece foldable acrylic IOL (Carlevale, ISP60VL) made of a combination of a hydrophilic and a hydrophobic polymer. It contains two plugs intended for transscleral fixation without the need for suturing [4, 7, 12].

Conclusion

While haptic- or suture externalization using forceps seems easier to learn, there are still difficulties to overcome with regard to the possible risk of breaking or deforming a haptic. With the combination of IOLs with PVDF haptic and a forceps-based approach, potential hurdles can be overcome easier than ever before. Despite of the surgical challenges in IOL exchange, IOL re-fixation or secondary IOL placement the instruments described above significantly reduce the challenges of scleral fixation techniques.

References

1. Agrawal V, Raju B. Creating the flange in Yamane's technique. Indian J Ophthalmol. 2021;69(2):465. https://www.ncbi.nlm.nih.gov/pmc/articles/PMC7933861/.
2. Ahn JK, Yu HG, Chung H, Wee WR, Lee J-H. Transscleral fixation of a foldable intraocular lens in aphakic vitrectomized eyes. J Cataract Refract Surg. 2003;29:2390. https://doi.org/10.1016/S0886-3350(03)00338-9.
3. Amon M, Bernhart C, Geitzenauer W, Kahraman G. The forceps-needle: combining needle and grasping functions in a single instrument. J Cataract Refract Surg. 2021;47:123–6. https://doi.org/10.1097/j.jcrs.0000000000000302.
4. Barca F, Caporossi T, de Angelis L, Giansanti F, Savastano A, Di Leo L, Rizzo S. Transscleral plugs fixated IOL: a new paradigm for sutureless scleral fixation. J Cataract Refract Surg. 2020;46:716. https://doi.org/10.1097/j.jcrs.0000000000000135.
5. Bergren RL. Four-point fixation technique for sutured posterior chamber intraocular lenses. Arch Ophthalmol. 1994;1960(112):1485–7. https://doi.org/10.1001/archopht.1994.01090230099029.
6. Canabrava S, Canêdo Domingos Lima AC, Ribeiro G. Four-flanged intrascleral intraocular lens fixation technique: no flaps, no knots, no glue. Cornea. 2020;39:527–8. https://doi.org/10.1097/ico.0000000000002185.
7. Carlà MM, Boselli F, Giannuzzi F, Caporossi T, Gambini G, Mosca L, Savastano A, Rizzo S. Sutureless scleral fixation Carlevale IOL: a review on the novel designed lens. Int Ophthalmol. 2022. https://doi.org/10.1007/s10792-022-02579-w.
8. Kahraman G, Amon M. New supplementary intraocular lens for refractive enhancement in pseudophakic patients. J Cataract Refract Surg. 2010;36:1090–4. https://doi.org/10.1016/j.jcrs.2009.12.045.
9. Ma KK, Yuan A, Sharifi S, Pineda R. A biomechanical study of flanged intrascleral haptic fixation of three-piece intraocular lenses. Am J Ophthalmol. 2021;227:45–52. https://doi.org/10.1016/j.ajo.2021.02.021.
10. Park CH, Lee SJ. Suture fixation technique for a single-piece foldable closed-loop intraocular lens. Korean J Ophthalmol KJO. 2008;22:205–9. https://doi.org/10.3341/kjo.2008.22.4.205.

11. Piercing Flanged Technique Durval Carvalho Jr-Winner World Webnar Cataract and Refractive Surgery, 2021.
12. Rossi T, Iannetta D, Romano V, Carlevale C, Forlini M, Telani S, Imburgia A, Mularoni A, Fontana L, Ripandelli G. A novel intraocular lens designed for sutureless scleral fixation: surgical series. Graefes Arch Clin Exp Ophthalmol. 2021;259:257–62. https://doi.org/10.1007/s00417-020-04789-3.
13. Sewelam A. Four-point fixation of posterior chamber intraocular lenses in children with unilateral aphakia. J Cataract Refract Surg. 2003;29:294–300. https://doi.org/10.1016/s0886-3350(02)01531-6.
14. Shen JF, Deng S, Hammersmith KM, Kuo AN, Li JY, Weikert MP, Shtein RM. Intraocular lens implantation in the absence of zonular support: an outcomes and safety update: a report by the American Academy of Ophthalmology. Ophthalmology. 2020;127:1234–58. https://doi.org/10.1016/j.ophtha.2020.03.005.
15. Vote BJ, Tranos P, Bunce C, Charteris DG, Da Cruz L. Long-term outcome of combined pars plana vitrectomy and scleral fixated sutured posterior chamber intraocular lens implantation. Am J Ophthalmol. 2006;141:308–12. https://doi.org/10.1016/j.ajo.2005.09.012.
16. Yamane S, Inoue M, Arakawa A, Kadonosono K. Sutureless 27-gauge needle-guided intrascleral intraocular lens implantation with lamellar scleral dissection. Ophthalmology. 2014;121:61–6. https://doi.org/10.1016/j.ophtha.2013.08.043.
17. Yamane S, Sato S, Maruyama-Inoue M, Kadonosono K. Flanged intrascleral intraocular lens fixation with double-needle technique. Ophthalmology. 2017;124:1136–42. https://doi.org/10.1016/j.ophtha.2017.03.036.

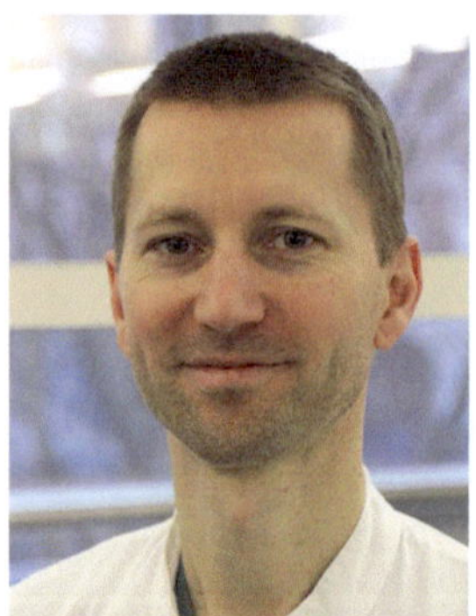

Wolfgang Geitzenauer, MD MSc FEBO graduated from the Medical University of Vienna, Austria and subsequently spent his ophthalmic residency at the Department of Ophthalmlogy. Due to his interest in research and clinical trials he acquired a Master's degree in Epidemiology from the London School of Hygiene and Tropical Medicine. After three years of fellowships in the United Kingdom (West of England Eye Unit, Exeter) he returned back to Vienna and has worked since at the St. John's Hospital as a consultant ophthalmic surgeon with his main interest in cataract and corneal diseases.

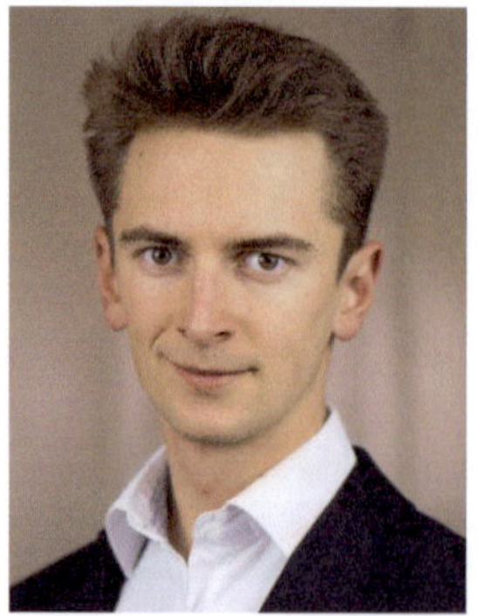

Konstantin Seiller-Tarbuk is an ophthalmologist from Vienna. Having studied at the Medical University of Vienna he is currently finishing his residency at the Hospital of St. John of God. In addition to his clinical work, Konstantin has actively engaged in teaching lessons and practical courses, sharing his knowledge and expertise with physicians, medical students and nursing professionals for many years. Additionally, he brings a unique and innovative perspective as a young doctor. In combination with his knowledge in video and photo editing, he is a valuable contributor to the book chapter, bringing insights and practical knowledge to the table.

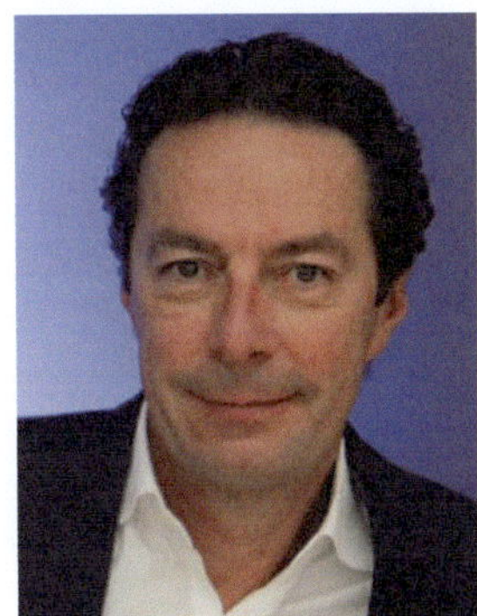

Michael Amon, MD is chairman of the Sigmund Freud Medical University and head of the eye department at the Academic Teaching Hospital of St. John Vienna. In 2009 he was awarded a professorship by the Medical University Vienna. He was Austrian delegate for EBO and UEMS, board-member and congress president of DGII, and president of the Austrian- and Viennese Ophthalmological Society. He was board-member of the ESCRS and is board-member of the Austrian Ophthalmological Society and head of the Austrian Cataract Committee. Since 2012 he is member of the Education Committee of the ESCRS. In a citation analysis in 2008 he was cited as 5th influential author in Europe and 20th worldwide. He is member of several editorial boards and of the IIIC. Beside different intraocular implants, he invented the first single-piece add-on IOL and different surgical instruments. With the development of the term 'uveal and capsular biocompatibility' he underlined his main scientific interest in IOLs and in cataract surgery in compromised eyes. He has performed over 30,000 intraocular procedures, including pediatric cataract-, posterior segment-, glaucoma- and corneal-surgery. He organised main-symposia, instructional courses and wet-labs, chaired sessions, presented on learning platforms and performed live surgery at international and national congresses.

Pearls from the Authors and Answers to Important Questions

Michael Amon

Abstract

Causes for decentration and for capsular alterations such as dead bag syndrome and Soemmerrings Ring will be discussed. The influence of IOL-material and IOL design on decentration or on capsular alteration will be described. Additionally in this chapter optimized procedures for flanging techniques will be shown. The authors describe their worst case and establish strategies to avoid complications. They share their most important pearls how to crate perfect results in scleral IOL-fixation. Finally the authors explain why and when they use their special technique, talk about contraindications for flanging techniques and state if they prefer haptic- or suture-flanging.

Keywords

Dead bag syndrome · Soemmerrings ring · IOL-decentration · Flanging techniques · IOL-material · IOL-design · IOL refixation · IOL exchange · Iridectomy · Vitrectomy · Optic-capture

Introduction

In this chapter the authors give tips and tricks in order to steepen the learning curve of flanging techniques for surgeons who want to start with these elegant techniques and for surgeons who want to improve their surgery and to enhance the surgical result.

M. Amon (✉)
Sigmund Freud Medical University, Vienna, Austria
e-mail: amon@augenchirurg.com

Department of Ophthalmology, Academic Teaching Hospital of St. John, Vienna, Austria

In this part we also collected answers from the experts to important questions in this field, in order to sum up this topic and in order to show that even different approaches may lead to our aim, the optimized surgical result.

I want to thank all of them for their wonderful contribution!

1. **Pearls how to optimize results in scleral IOL-fixation and how to avoid complications:**

Shin Yamane

1. The positional relationship of the wounds; It is appropriate for the wound where the IOL is inserted and the left sclerotomy for haptic fixation to be in positions that are separated by approximately 70°. By keeping this positional relationship, the haptic and the needle can be aligned.
2. Double needle technique: Placing the leading haptic in the inner cavity of the 30-gauge needle makes the positional relationship of the trailing haptic and the second 30-gauge needle appropriate and facilitates easy insertion. If the leading haptic is pulled out together with the 30-gauge needle, the IOL will rotate in the counterclockwise direction. It is difficult to insert the tip of the trailing haptic into a 30-gauge needle in this situation.
3. The insertion angle of the 30-gauge needle; In order to avoid IOL tilt and dislocation, the haptics must be fixed symmetrically. Needle stabilizer is useful to make insertion angle constant.
4. Making and fixation of flange; The cautery should not touch the haptic while cauterization to avoid adhesion. The haptic should be dry to avoid twisted flange. The appropriate length of the haptic to cauterize is 0.5 to 1.0 mm. The flange must be fixed completely inside the sclera. If not, the flange may move under conjunctiva. If the size of the flange was too large to insert into the scleral tunnel, the entry site of the scleral tunnel should be enlarged using 30-gauge needle.

Sérgio Canabrava

1. careful choice of the material used: for 5-0 polypropylene, the best needle is the 27G insulin needle, whereas 6-0 polypropylene suture requires 29G insulin needle;
2. mark 2 mm from the limbus and create a long scleral tunnel that is parallel to the limbus and about 2 mm long;
3. increase the tension of the polypropylene suture by holding its base with the 23-gauge micro forceps in close apposition to the sclera
4. the polypropylene suture should be cut 1.2–1.5 mm from the micro forceps;

5. make sure that the flange is completely buried within the scleral tunnel at the end of the surgery;

Ehud Assia, Avner Belkin

1. Prolene 6-0 suture (inserted through 29G or 30G needle) is an optimal compromise of suture thickness. It does not biodegradate and is user friendly and easy to manipulate.
2. Make sure the flange is covered by both conjunctiva and tenon, not just the conjunctiva
3. Intrastromal flange may dislocate into the vitreous cavity. Do not overstretch the suture during fixation.
4. Transoptic fixation by threading a needle through the lens material is a valid and effective option, however the suture may cheese-wire through the lens. Careful surgery is then required with minimal stress on the suture.
5. Tilt and decentration, occasionally seen following 2-point fixation, can be effectively treated by adding 1–2 fixation points (including trans optic)

Michael Amon

1. If you need an infusion, use a scleral port. The anterior chamber is less crowded then. Especially for an IOL exchange the posterior to anterior current is helpful for the removal of capsular remnants.
2. Try to float capsular remnants out through the main incision as grasping or cutting and aspiration is not possible sometimes.
3. Utilize the scleral port for a very controlled pars plana vitrectomy.
4. Avoid to traumatize the iris root during scleral tunnel preparation. Do not perforate too anterior.
5. Use PVDF haptics for the Yamane technique as they are more flexible and warranty better memory.
6. Avoid collapse of the anterior chamber by thorough titration of the infusion pressure. Treat a posterior blockage with vitrectomy posterior to the IOL/capsule compartment.
7. The forceps-needle is helpful for the externalization of haptics or sutures. You can grasp the material at a suboptimal angle and you will not lose the grasped material.
8. An undamaged IOL can be re-fixated in some cases. You do avoid the main incision, and create less surgical trauma and less risk of a biometrical surprise.
9. Primary shortening of polypropylene sutures to a few centimeters makes manipulation easier. For double flanged suture fixation, after flanging of the second suture, it is intended that the suture is under moderate tension. So the suture end slides behind the conjunctiva and Tenons layer by itself and stops right at the scleral tunnel.

10. Low temperature cautery creates a better control during the flanging process.

Gabor Scharioth

1. cilliary sulcus sclerotomy
   Use 23G cannula placed on a syringe with Luer look, place around 2 mm postlimbal, observe iris, if iris root moves just create a new sclerotomy 0.5 mm posterior, some eyes have a relatively posterior AC angle (anterior limbus, small cornea, high myopes etc.), direct cannula towards center of the eye, flat insertion increases risk for iris damage, place sclerotomies exactly 180° from each other, corneal marking of 180° might be useful.
2. limbusparallel intrascleral tunnel with 23G cannula or 23G MVR blade
   Use new 23 G cannula, start from inside the sclerotomy, stay limbusparallel, externalize tip of cannula after 2 mm.
3. vitrectomy
   Deep anterior or pars plana vitrectomy.
4. capsulectomy
   There is no advantage of leaving capsule remnants, they might cause IOL tilt or decentration, posterior synechiae etc.
5. continuous infusion (AC maintainer or pars plana)
   This keeps the eye firm for easier manipulations, OVD would be lost into vitreous cavity and cause postop IOP spike.
6. intrascleral haptic fixation
   Ensure complete intrascleral fixation, that prevents late erosion, haptic end can be flanged or bented to prevent slippage (esp. in young patients, high myopes with elastic and/or thin sclera).
7. proper instrumentation
   Scharioth forceps, DORC.
   Combination of straight and bent forceps improves manipulations, straight forceps also useful to lift a luxated IOL from retina, curved forceps esp. in deep seated eyes and/or patients with big nose and/or eye brow useful.
   Small gauge 25G (or 27G) forceps preferable, serrated forceps is a good alternative.
8. in case of leackage suture sclerotomies
   Vicryl 8 × 0 sutures.
9. reverse pupillary block and iris capture
   Perform peripheral iridectomy with small gauge vitrectome, in recurrent iris capture use pilocarpine eye drops for at least six months.

2. Answers from the authors to important questions

2.a. Preop condition

What are the most frequent causes for IOL-dislocation or for insufficient capsular support?

Liliana Werner: Early postoperative intraocular lens (IOL) dislocation (occurring less than 3 months postoperatively) is usually secondary to poor IOL fixation. Late postoperative IOL dislocation (occurring 3 months or more after surgery) is usually a result of zonular weakness. Major risk factors for zonulysis and late in-the-bag IOL dislocation include trauma and conditions leading to progressive zonular weakness, such as pseudoexfoliation (PEX) syndrome (considered the most common risk factor), high myopia, uveitis, as well as certain connective tissue disorders (Marfan's syndrome, homocystinuria, hyperlysinemia, Ehlers-Danlos syndrome, scleroderma, and Weil-Marchesani's syndrome). Zonular weakness may also be observed after vitreoretinal surgery; zonules also become more friable as patients age, especially in PEX patients.

Shin Yamane: IOL dislocation of unknown cause

Sergio Canabrava: Post-Phaco

Ehud Assia: pseudoexfoliation, high myopia, blunt trauma, advanced age, aggressive surgery, congenital connective tissue anomalies

Michael Amon: PEX

Are there any predictors for the development of Soemmering's ring formation or for the development of the dead bag syndrome?

Liliana Werner: Soemmering's ring formation depends in part, on how well the capsular bag was evacuated during surgery. If a lot of residual cortical material and lens epithelial cells (LECs) are left behind, the chances for more Soemmering's ring formation are higher. Younger people also have tendency for more Soemmering's ring formation, and therefore more posterior capsule opacification (PCO).

For the dead bag syndrome, there are still a lot of unknowns, so clear predictors could still not be identified. When looking at the results of our first peer-reviewed study on this syndrome, especially regarding the scarcity of LECs in the capsules, many surgeons are naturally asking the question whether capsular polishing has any relationship with this syndrome. However, no clear association between polishing and dead bag syndrome could be established so far.

Shin Yamane: No

Sergio Canabrava: I don't have experience with

Ehud Assia: Sommering's ring occurs more frequently in younger age and following incomplete removal of lens material. There are still no clues for the development of Dead Bag Syndrome.

Is there a correlation of the kind of capsular alteration with type of the IOL?
Liliana Werner: As you will see in the answer below, in analyses of pseudophakic eyes obtained postmortem, as well as clinical studies, plate–haptic silicone IOLs have been associated with an increased risk for anterior capsule opacification (ACO) with secondary capsule contraction, which may subsequently increase the risk for dislocation.

Shin Yamane: An IOL with a rim is less prone to anterior capsular contraction.

Ehud Assia: lens material, square edge, haptic angulation, total diameter and lens design were all shown decades ago to affect capsular behavior. Separation of the anterior and posterior capsules by a thick lens or a ring was shown to significantly reduce capsular opacification.

Is there a correlation of the frequency of IOL-dislocation or of zonular defects with the type of IOL?
Liliana Werner: In a 2021 review paper on late in-the-bag IOL dislocation (Kristianslund O, Dalby M, Drolsum L. Late in-the-bag intraocular lens dislocation. J Cataract Refract Surg. 2021 Jul 1;47(7):942–954), the authors reported that some of the studies included in the review have indicated a possible association between dislocation of the IOL-capsular bag complex and certain IOL designs and materials. However, the results were inconsistent, and when associations were found, they likely reflected the IOL types most frequently used in the years preceding the corresponding studies. In analyses of pseudophakic eyes obtained postmortem, as well as clinical studies, plate–haptic silicone IOLs have been associated with an increased risk for anterior capsule opacification (ACO) with secondary capsule contraction, which may subsequently increase the risk for dislocation.

Shin Yamane: No

Ehud Assia: not to my knowledge.

What are the causes for the dead bag syndrome?
Liliana Werner: The term dead bag syndrome is used to describe cases where the capsular bag itself apparently becomes diaphanous and floppy, and unable to support the IOL within it. The common feature among these cases appears to be the presence of a very clear capsular bag many years after surgery. At presentation, there may be subluxation of the IOL inside of the floppy bag, sometimes through a peripheral capsular defect, while the capsular bag itself is still centered. In other cases, there may be late in-the-bag IOL dislocation. This syndrome does not appear to have any association with a particular IOL design or material, nor with intraoperative capsular polishing. The exact etiology of dead bag syndrome is still unknown. The initial problem may be in the residual LECs, or in the capsule itself. The main feature of histopathological analyses of available explanted capsular bags so far is capsular splitting or delamination, and we believe late postoperative zonular failure is related to capsule splitting/delamination occurring at the level of zonular attachments.

Shin Yamane: Don't know.

Ehud Assia: Time after surgery (typically over 15 years) characterizes almost all cases of DBS. The syndrome was reported with all types of lens materials (hydrophobic, hydrophilic and silicone) and the operations are usually uneventful.

Do dislocated IOLs in capsular bags with dead bag syndrome show less damage than IOLs in those with Soemmering's ring?
Liliana Werner: In the specimens received in our lab, represented by in-the-bag dislocated IOLs, there is usually not much damage to the IOLs per se

Shin Yamane: Yes

Ehud Assia: Dead bag syndrome usually relates to capsular breaks with no apparent living cells. It is questionable whether zonular defects and residual Sommering's ring are part of this syndrome.

Which kind of IOL damage is most common in your IOL-samples after explantation?
Liliana Werner: After explantation, there may be findings such as scratches, broken haptics, cuts or such, pigmentary dispersion; nothing very specific and likely related to the explantation procedure itself

Shin Yamane: Variants of Haptics

Ehud Assia: Lens material opacification (i.e. calcification of hydrophillic lenses)

Michael Amon: we sometimes find bent IOL-haptics with total loss of their memory, sometimes YAG-pits, sometimes foreign-body giant cells and pigment on the IOL surface.

2.b. **Surgery**

Do you stop anticoagulation before flanging surgery?
Shin Yamane: No

Sergio Canabrava: Yes

Ehud Assia: never

Michael Amon: No.

Which kind of anesthesia do you prefer?
Shin Yamane: Sub Tenon anesthesia

Sergio Canabrava: Peribulbar

Ehud Assia: topical (drops) and intracameral (combined)

Michael Amon: peribulbar or general anesthesia.

In your routine cases do you use OVDs only, anterior chamber maintainer or a scleral port only, or do you combine OVD with infusion?
Shin Yamane: OVD with infusion

Sergio Canabrava: Posterior maintainer

Ehud Assia: I combine OVD (if and whenever needed) with ACM

Michael Amon: scleral port for exchange and for IOL implantation, OVD for easy refixation cases. Combination sometimes.

Do you perform vitrectomy in all cases and which type of vitrectomy do you use?
Shin Yamane: Pars plana vitrectomy for all cases

Sergio Canabrava: All scleral fixation cases. Posterior Vitrectomy

Michael Amon: Thorough anterior vitrectomy utilizing the scleral port. Posterior VE for cases with IOLs luxated to the posterior pole. No VE for simple refixation of a CTR/IOL complex.

In which case do you perform an iridectomy?
Shin Yamane: Cases without small pupil

Sergio Canabrava: None

Ehud Assia: Only with AC-IOL

Michael Amon: never intraoperatively.

What is your strategy in the case of an optic capture?
Shin Yamane: Pilocarpine eye drops and pupiloplasty

Ehud Assia: In many cases no surgical intervention is required. It annoys the surgeon more than affects the patient. Surgical intervention depends on the underlying cause

Michael Amon: YAG iridotomy in case of IOL capture, initial mydriasis followed by miotic treatment, surgical reintervention or keep it, if no problems.

In the case of a clinically significant tilt or decentration, what is your approach?
Shin Yamane: Refixation or IOL exchange

Sergio Canabrava: Back to operating room

Ehud Assia: I usually add a fixation point by scleral or iris fixation, including suturing the fibrosed capsule to the sclera

Michael Amon: surgical reintervention, 3-point fixation.

What is your strategy in the case of a conjunctival erosion of a flange?
Shin Yamane: Enlarge the scleral tunnel to embed the flange into the sclera

Sergio Canabrava: Back to operate room

Ehud Assia: The flange MUST be covered. The conjunctiva and tenon are released around the flange and sutured above it

Michael Amon: 1. Intervention at the slitlamp: pressing flange into distal scleral tunnel. 2. Surgical intervention: opening distal scleral tunnel, scleral flap or patch in rare cases with very thin sclera.

Is your limbal distance for IOL-fixation always the same?
Shin Yamane: Yes

Sergio Canabrava: Yes. 2 mm

Ehud Assia: usually 1.5–2.0 mm from the anatomical limbus

Michael Amon: 2 mm from the limbus. In cases of refixation posterior incision 2.5 mm, radial, anterior incision 1.5–2.0 mm.

Do you also use alternative solutions for an IOL-fixation to scleral flanging?
Shin Yamane: No

Sergio Canabrava: Yes. Glasses

Ehud Assia: Yes!, prolene 9-0 suture is effective and does not break, and is used in cases of additional fixation. Also iris fixation is an excellent option (prolene 9-0)

Michael Amon: Only in cases with severe scleral pathology. Then I perform posterior iris-fixation.

Haptic- or suture flanging, what is your preference and why?
Shin Yamane: Haptic flanging. We have no IOL with closed loop haptic in our country

Sergio Canabrava: Double Flanged Polypropylene, because my preference is 4 Flanged with 4 flanged points

Ehud Assia: definitely suture flanging. Haptic flanging is done with the IOL already in the posterior segment, requires good visualization and is associated with numerous complications. Suture flanging is safer, more convenient, can provide more than 2-point fixation and results are excellent

Michael Amon: Yamane technique for aphakia and after IOL exchange, double flanged sutures for refixation of CTRs or IOLs with closed loops.

Are there any contraindications for flanging techniques?
Shin Yamane: Collagen disease that causes scleritis

Sergio Canabrava: Yes. Thin sclera

Ehud Assia: not really, we successfully used flanging fixation also in high myopes, thin sclera in megaloglobus, Marfans etc.

Michael Amon: severe scleral pathologies such as anterior staphyloma.

Do you always exchange dislocated IOLs or do you re-fixate the IOL sometimes?
Shin Yamane: Exchange

Sergio Canabrava: Depends of the situation

Ehud Assia: my primary preference is to re-fixate the same IOL. The lens is good. The problem is the malposition therefore the logical solution is to reposition

Michael Amon: If the IOL has no evident damage, I prefer re-fixation. With this technique I avoid a main incision and can expect a good biometrical result.

What was your worst experience with your flanging technique?
Shin Yamane: Ciliary body dialysis

Sergio Canabrava: Patient with full retinal detachment

Ehud Assia: repeated decentration and tilt following various flanging techniques. Required 4 operation to finally stabilize the IOL

Michael Amon: I accidently damaged the trailing haptic with cautery, and had to exchange the already implanted, flanged IOL.

Would you expect breakage due to biodegradation of haptics or sutures in the long term?
Shin Yamane: No.

Sergio Canabrava: Till now, not!

Ehud Assia: 5-0 to 7-0 prolene sutures—no chance.

Michael Amon: Because of the dimension (mainly 6-0 polypropylene) I do not expect. Till now no case.

Do we need better implants for flanging techniques?
Shin Yamane: We need better IOL

Ehud Assia: absolutely yes, designed for 4-point fixation

Michael Amon: there exists a wide spectrum of IOLs on the market already, but yes, IOLs made for 4-point flanged suture fixation (loops with 4 eyelets).

How can we steepen the learning curve?
Shin Yamane: Use SimulEye

Sergio Canabrava: Wetlabs

Ehud Assia: practice makes perfect! Simple artificial eyes or cadaveric sheep, goat and cow eyes are excellent for training

Michael Amon: wetlabs, watching videos, a lot of practice.

Are flanging techniques a good option for refractive rehabilitation?
Shin Yamane: Yes.

Sergio Canabrava: Yes.

Ehud Assia: I believe they are currently the best option.

Michael Amon: Yes, the best option.

Are flanging techniques an option for less experienced surgeons?
Shin Yamane: No

Sergio Canabrava: I don't suggest any scleral fixation technique for less experienced surgeons

Ehud Assia: yes, but practice in a lab is required

Michael Amon: experienced surgeons only, but with hard work most surgeons may become experienced

In case of intraoperative loss of the capsular bag, how would you proceed with your surgery?

1. Stop surgery and perform a second intervention.
   Sergio Canabrava.
2. Proceed, but switch to a different kind of anesthesia.
   Shin Yamane: Add sub Tenon anesthesia, Flange a 3-piece IOL with PVDF haptics.

   Michael Amon: in a calm surgical situation I proceed or switch to peribulbar anesthesia and flange a 3-piece IOL, in a stressed situation I stop after anterior vitrectomy and postpone for a second intervention.
3. Proceed and flange an IOL or use another fixation technique (IOL type).
   Ehud Assia.

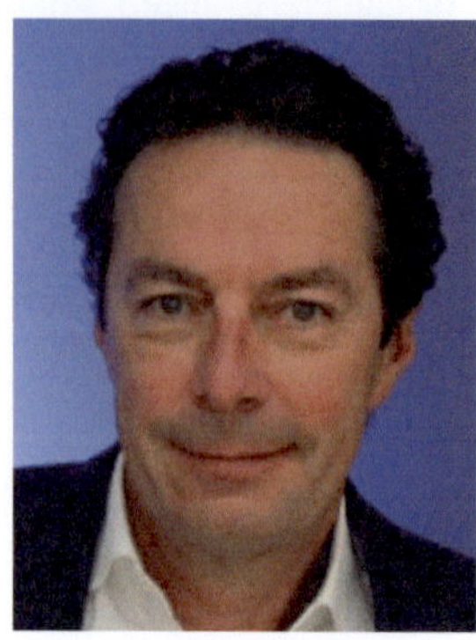

Michael Amon MD is chairman of the Sigmund Freud Medical University and head of the eye department at the Academic Teaching Hospital of St. John Vienna. In 2009 he was awarded a professorship by the Medical University Vienna. He was Austrian delegate for EBO and UEMS, board-member and congress president of DGII, and president of the Austrian- and Viennese Ophthalmological Society. He was board-member of the ESCRS and is board-member of the Austrian Ophthalmological Society and head of the Austrian Cataract Committee. Since 2012 he is member of the Education Committee of the ESCRS. In a citation analysis in 2008 he was cited as 5th influential author in Europe and 20th worldwide. He is member of several editorial boards and of the IIIC. Beside different intraocular implants, he invented the first single-piece add-on IOL and different surgical instruments. With the development of the term 'uveal and capsular biocompatibility' he underlined his main scientific interest in IOLs and in cataract surgery in compromised eyes. He has performed over 30,000 intraocular procedures, including pediatric cataract-, posterior segment-, glaucoma- and corneal-surgery. He organised main-symposia, instructional courses and wet-labs, chaired sessions, presented on learning platforms and performed live surgery at international and national congresses.